The Complete Diabetic Cookbook for Beginners

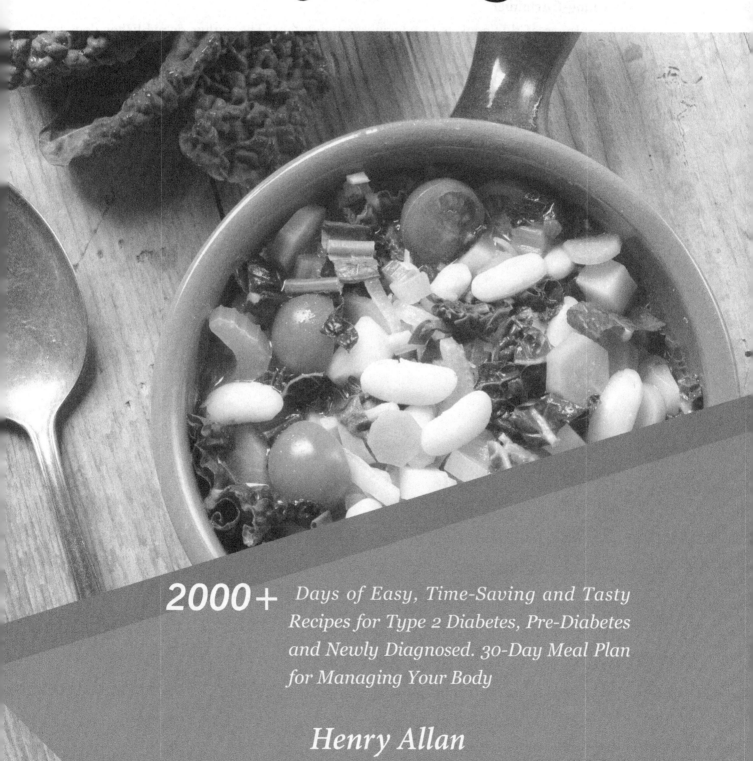

2000+ Days of Easy, Time-Saving and Tasty Recipes for Type 2 Diabetes, Pre-Diabetes and Newly Diagnosed. 30-Day Meal Plan for Managing Your Body

Henry Allan

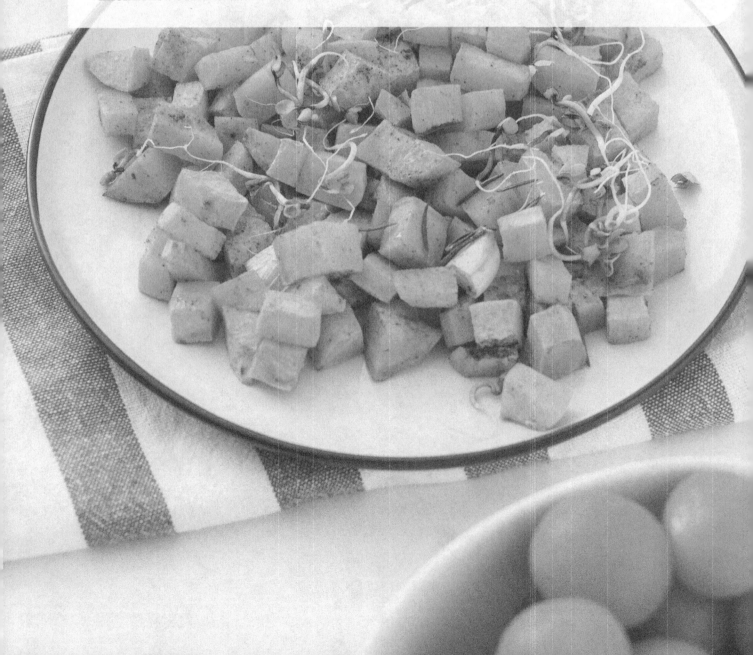

Table of Contents

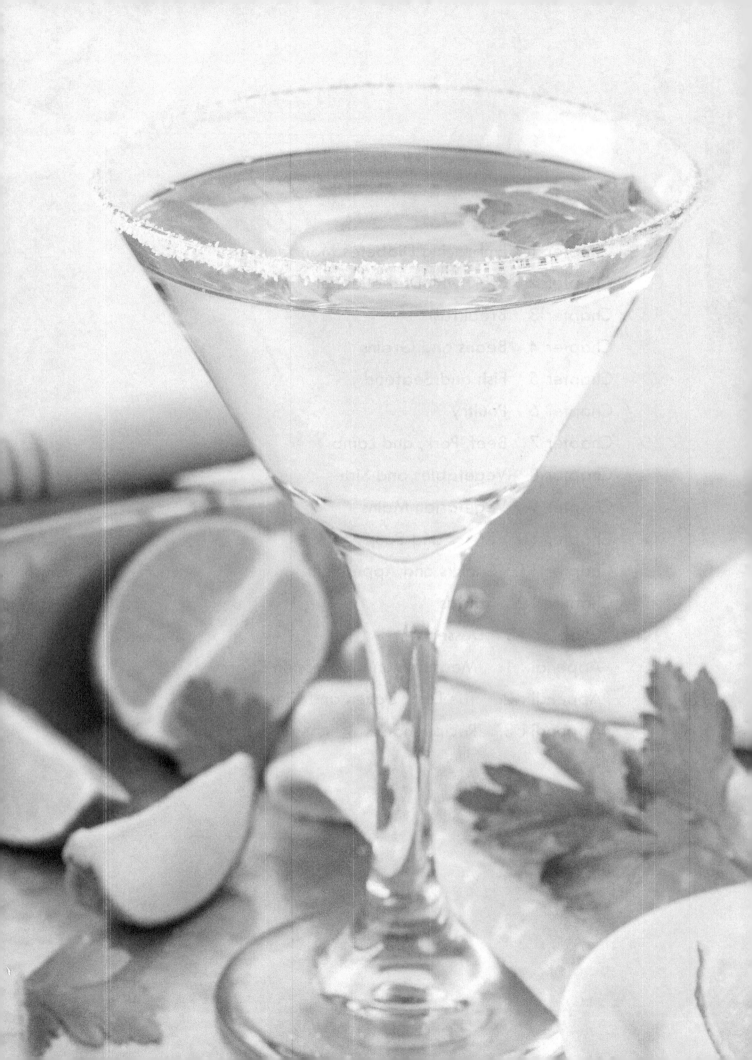

INTRODUCTION

Welcome to the Diabetic Cookbook, a culinary journey designed to empower individuals living with diabetes to savor delicious, nourishing meals while maintaining stable blood sugar levels and overall well-being. This cookbook is a testament to the belief that diabetes management doesn't have to compromise the pleasure of eating. Instead, it invites you to discover a world of flavor, creativity, and balance, all while keeping your health in mind.

Living with diabetes can be challenging, but it's crucial to remember that a diagnosis doesn't mean you have to sacrifice the joy of eating. With the right knowledge and approach, you can still enjoy a wide array of wholesome and satisfying dishes. This cookbook is specially curated to help you navigate the realm of diabetes-friendly cooking, offering a diverse selection of recipes that cater to different tastes, dietary needs, and culinary preferences.

Throughout these pages, you'll find a treasure trove of recipes that embrace fresh, whole ingredients and strike a harmonious balance between nutrients. From hearty breakfasts to delectable desserts, each recipe is crafted to not only delight your taste buds but also support your body's health requirements. We understand that maintaining stable blood sugar levels is crucial, so rest assured that each dish includes nutritional information and portion guidance to help you make informed choices.

In addition to the recipes themselves, this cookbook is a valuable resource for understanding the principles of diabetic-friendly cooking. We'll explore smart ingredient substitutions, portion control, and mindful eating habits that can enhance your diabetes management journey. Empowered with this knowledge, you'll be better equipped to tailor your meals to your specific needs and preferences.

Whether you're newly diagnosed with diabetes or have been living with it for years, this cookbook is here to inspire and guide you towards a more vibrant and fulfilling life. It's time to break free from the notion that diabetes means restriction, and instead, embrace the vast array of culinary possibilities available to you.

So, let's embark on this flavorful adventure together, celebrating food, health, and the joy of cooking. Let the Diabetic Cookbook be your trusted companion, supporting you in making informed choices that lead to a happier, healthier you. Remember, managing diabetes can be a positive and empowering journey, and it all begins with the choices you make in the kitchen.

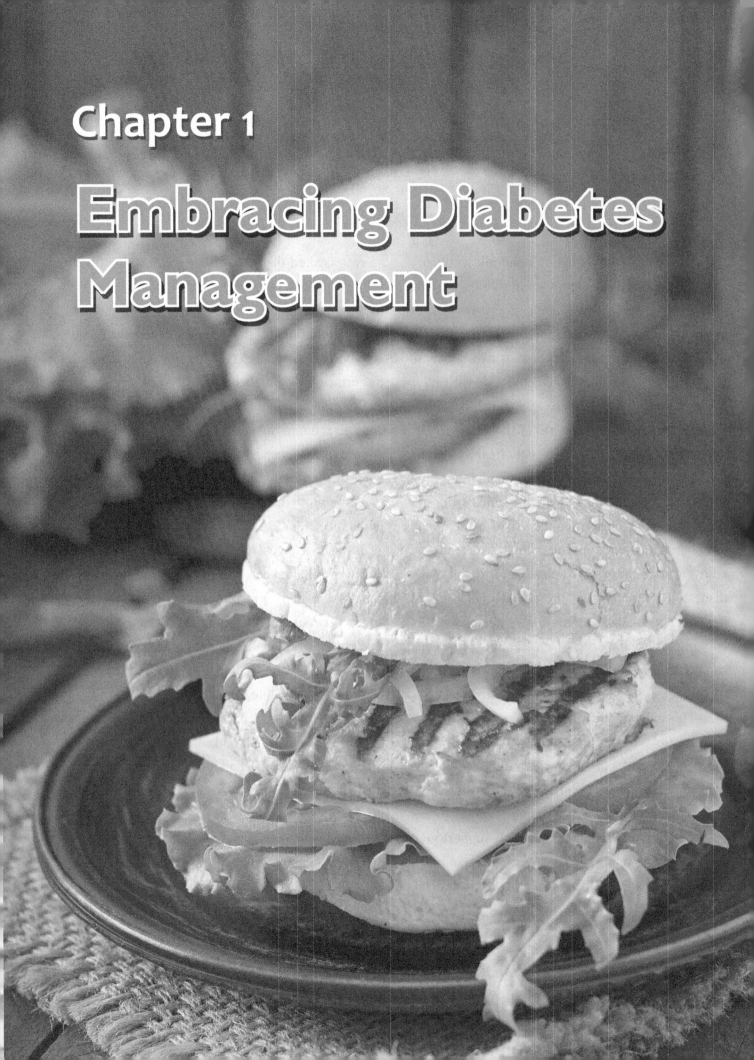

Chapter 1
Embracing Diabetes Management

Definition of Diabetic Diet

The Diabetic Diet, also known as Medical Nutrition Therapy (MNT) for diabetes, is a specialized eating plan designed to help individuals with diabetes manage their blood sugar levels effectively. This diet emphasizes balanced nutrition, portion control, and making thoughtful food choices to maintain stable glucose levels and promote overall health.

The primary goals of a diabetic diet are:

Blood Sugar Regulation: The main objective of the diabetic diet is to manage blood sugar levels within a healthy range. This is achieved by controlling the intake of carbohydrates, as they have the most significant impact on blood sugar levels. By spreading carbohydrate consumption throughout the day and combining them with protein and healthy fats, the body can better regulate the rise and fall of blood glucose levels.

Weight Management: For individuals with diabetes, achieving and maintaining a healthy weight is vital. Excess body weight can make it more challenging to control blood sugar levels, and losing weight can often improve insulin sensitivity and reduce the need for diabetes medications.

Cardiovascular Health: Diabetes is associated with an increased risk of cardiovascular diseases. A diabetic diet aims to reduce the intake of saturated and trans fats while promoting the consumption of heart-healthy fats, fiber, and plant-based foods to support cardiovascular health.

Maintaining Optimal Nutrition: The diabetic diet is not about deprivation; it's about making smart and informed choices. It focuses on including nutrient-dense foods such as whole grains, fruits, vegetables, lean proteins, and low-fat dairy, ensuring that individuals with diabetes receive all essential vitamins, minerals, and other nutrients.

Key components of the diabetic diet include:

Carbohydrate Management: Carbohydrates directly impact blood sugar levels, so managing their intake is crucial. The diabetic diet emphasizes complex carbohydrates with a lower glycemic index (GI), as they cause a slower and steadier rise in blood glucose levels. It also encourages portion control to prevent blood sugar spikes.

Healthy Fats: The diet promotes the consumption of heart-healthy fats, such as those found in avocados, nuts, seeds, and olive oil, while limiting saturated and trans fats, often found in processed and fried foods.

Protein: Including adequate protein in the diet helps stabilize blood sugar levels, supports muscle health, and promotes satiety. Sources of lean protein, such as poultry, fish, tofu, and legumes, are recommended.

Fiber-rich Foods: Foods high in dietary fiber, like whole grains, fruits, vegetables, and legumes, can slow down the absorption of glucose, leading to more stable blood sugar levels and improved digestive health.

Regular Meal Timing: Consistency in meal timing is essential for individuals with diabetes. Eating at regular intervals helps maintain consistent blood sugar levels throughout the day.

It's essential to remember that each person's diabetic diet should be tailored to their individual health needs, lifestyle, and personal preferences. Working with a registered dietitian or healthcare professional experienced in diabetes management can be immensely helpful in creating a personalized meal plan that aligns with specific goals and requirements. Additionally, regular monitoring of blood sugar levels and adjustments to the diet can further optimize diabetes management and overall well-being.

Importance of Diabetes Management

Diabetes management plays a critical role in the overall health and well-being of individuals living with diabetes. It involves a combination of lifestyle changes, medication, and regular monitoring to keep blood sugar levels within a healthy range. The importance of diabetes management cannot be overstated, and here are some key reasons why it is essential:

Blood Sugar Control: The primary goal of diabetes management is to maintain stable blood sugar levels. Uncontrolled diabetes can lead to consistently high blood glucose levels, which, over time, can cause damage to blood vessels, nerves, and organs. Proper diabetes management helps prevent or delay the onset of diabetes-related complications such as heart disease, kidney disease, nerve damage, and vision problems.

Quality of Life: Effective diabetes management can significantly improve the quality of life for individuals with diabetes. By keeping blood sugar levels in check, they can avoid frequent fluctuations that may cause fatigue, irritability, and difficulty concentrating. Well-managed diabetes allows individuals to lead an active and fulfilling life without being limited by the condition.

Preventing Hypoglycemia: Diabetes management also involves preventing episodes of hypoglycemia (low blood sugar). Hypoglycemia can lead to dizziness, confusion, loss of consciousness, and, in severe cases, even life-threatening emergencies. By balancing medication, diet, and physical activity, individuals can minimize the risk of hypoglycemia.

Preventing Hyperglycemia: On the other end of the spectrum, diabetes management aims to prevent hyperglycemia (high blood sugar). Consistently high blood sugar levels can lead to a condition called diabetic ketoacidosis (DKA), which is a medical emergency requiring immediate treatment. Proper diabetes management helps avoid such dangerous situations.

Reducing the Need for Medications: Lifestyle changes, including a healthy diet, regular exercise, and weight management, can often reduce the need for diabetes medications or insulin. Some individuals may even achieve diabetes remission through effective management, especially in cases of type 2 diabetes.

Promoting Cardiovascular Health: Diabetes is a risk factor for cardiovascular diseases such as heart attacks and strokes. By managing diabetes, individuals can improve their cardiovascular health and reduce the risk of these serious complications.

Supporting Overall Health: Diabetes management is not just about controlling blood sugar levels; it also encourages overall health. A well-balanced diet, regular exercise, and other healthy habits promoted in diabetes management can lead to improved immune function, better weight management, and reduced risks of other chronic diseases.

Empowerment and Education: Engaging in diabetes management empowers individuals to take an active role in their health. Through education and awareness about diabetes and its management, individuals can make informed decisions and better navigate their daily lives with the condition.

In conclusion, diabetes management is essential for achieving optimal health outcomes and preventing complications associated with diabetes. A comprehensive approach that includes regular medical check-ups, a balanced diet, physical activity, and adherence to prescribed medications can significantly improve the overall well-being and longevity of individuals living with diabetes.

Breaking Myths and Stereotypes

Breaking myths and stereotypes surrounding diabetes is essential to provide accurate information, dispel misconceptions, and promote a more empathetic and informed understanding of the condition. Here are some common myths and stereotypes about diabetes, along with the truths that help break them:

1. Myth: Diabetes is caused by consuming too much sugar.

Truth: While excessive sugar consumption can contribute to weight gain and increase the risk of developing type 2 diabetes, it is not the sole cause. Type 1 diabetes is an autoimmune condition, and type 2 diabetes is influenced by various factors, including genetics, lifestyle, and obesity.

2. Myth: People with diabetes can't eat sweets or enjoy desserts.

Truth: Individuals with diabetes can enjoy sweets and desserts in moderation as part of a balanced diet. With careful carbohydrate counting and portion control, they can incorporate occasional treats without compromising their blood sugar levels.

3. Myth: Diabetes is only a "mild" condition that doesn't require serious attention.

Truth: Diabetes is a chronic medical condition that requires ongoing management and can lead to severe complications if not properly controlled. It demands constant monitoring of blood sugar levels, lifestyle adjustments, and, in some cases, medication or insulin.

4. Myth: People with diabetes can't participate in physical activities or exercise.

Truth: Regular physical activity is beneficial for individuals with diabetes. Exercise can improve insulin sensitivity, aid in weight management, and promote overall health. However, it's essential to consult healthcare professionals and tailor exercise routines to individual needs and limitations.

5. Myth: Only older people develop diabetes.

Truth: While age can be a risk factor for type 2 diabetes, diabetes can affect people of all ages, including children and young adults. Type 1 diabetes, in particular, often develops in childhood or early adulthood.

6. Myth: Insulin is a last resort and means diabetes is getting worse.

Truth: Insulin is a vital and sometimes necessary treatment for both type 1 and type 2 diabetes. It is not a sign of failure but rather a tool to manage blood sugar levels effectively and prevent complications.

7. Myth: Diabetes is contagious.

Truth: Diabetes is not contagious; it cannot be transmitted from one person to another through contact or any means of exposure.

8. Myth: People with diabetes are to blame for their condition.

Truth: Diabetes is a complex condition influenced by multiple factors, including genetics and lifestyle. Blaming individuals with diabetes for their condition perpetuates stigma and fails to recognize the diverse and unique factors that contribute to the development of the disease.

9. Myth: Diabetes can be cured by natural remedies or "superfoods."

Truth: While a healthy diet and lifestyle play a crucial role in diabetes management, there is no cure for diabetes. While certain foods may help manage blood sugar levels, they cannot eliminate the condition entirely.

Breaking these myths and stereotypes helps foster a more compassionate and supportive environment for individuals living with diabetes. It encourages accurate information dissemination, promotes early diagnosis, and encourages proactive diabetes management to prevent complications and improve overall well-being.

Understanding Nutritional Information

Understanding nutritional information is a fundamental aspect of making informed and healthy food choices. Nutritional information is typically provided on food labels and includes various key components that help individuals assess the nutrient content of a particular food product. Here are the essential elements of nutritional information and their significance:

Serving Size: The serving size indicates the recommended portion of the food product. All the nutritional values listed on the label are based on this specific serving size. It is crucial to pay attention to the serving size, as consuming more significant portions than recommended will result in higher nutrient intake.

Calories: Calories represent the amount of energy provided by the food per serving size. Understanding the calorie content is essential for weight management and maintaining a balanced diet.

Total Fat: This category provides information on the total amount of fat (in grams) per serving. It is further divided into subcategories: saturated fat, trans fat, and sometimes monounsaturated and polyunsaturated fats. Limiting the intake of saturated and trans fats is important for heart health, while incorporating healthy fats, like monounsaturated and polyunsaturated fats, is beneficial.

Cholesterol: Cholesterol content is given in milligrams and indicates the amount of cholesterol present in the food. High cholesterol intake can impact heart health, so it's essential to be mindful of its presence in food products.

Sodium: Sodium content is listed in milligrams and informs consumers about the amount of salt in the food. Monitoring sodium intake is essential for individuals with high blood pressure and heart conditions, as excess sodium can contribute to hypertension.

Total Carbohydrates: This category includes the total carbohydrates in grams, which consist of dietary fiber, sugars, and sometimes sugar alcohols. For individuals with diabetes, understanding the breakdown of carbohydrates can be crucial for managing blood sugar levels.

Dietary Fiber: Dietary fiber is a type of carbohydrate that is not fully digested by the body. It aids in digestion, helps regulate blood sugar levels, and promotes a feeling of fullness.

Total Sugars: Total sugars represent the sum of naturally occurring sugars (e.g., in fruits) and added sugars (e.g., sucrose or high-fructose corn syrup). Limiting added sugars in the diet is important for overall health, as excessive sugar intake can lead to various health issues.

Protein: Protein content is given in grams and represents the amount of protein present in the food. Protein is essential for building and repairing tissues and plays a vital role in various bodily functions.

Vitamins and Minerals: Some food labels provide information on specific vitamins and minerals present in the product, such as vitamin A, vitamin C, calcium, and iron. These nutrients are essential for various physiological processes in the body.

Understanding nutritional information empowers individuals to make healthier food choices that align with their dietary goals, health conditions, and nutritional needs. Reading food labels and comparing different products can help consumers make more informed decisions to support their overall well-being.

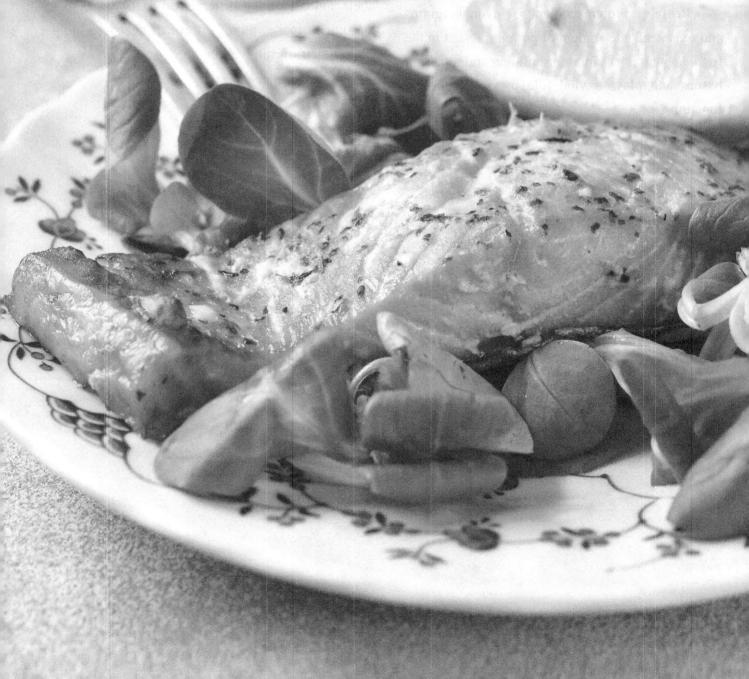

Chapter 2

Start with Diabetic Diet

Frequently Asked Questions

1. What is diabetes?

Diabetes is a chronic medical condition characterized by high blood sugar levels, either due to inadequate insulin production (Type 1 diabetes) or ineffective use of insulin by the body (Type 2 diabetes). It can lead to various complications if not managed properly.

2. How is diabetes diagnosed?

Diabetes is typically diagnosed through blood tests that measure blood glucose levels. Fasting blood glucose, oral glucose tolerance test, and hemoglobin A1c (HbA1c) are common tests used to diagnose diabetes.

3. What are the main types of diabetes?

The main types of diabetes are Type 1 diabetes, Type 2 diabetes, and gestational diabetes. Type 1 diabetes is an autoimmune condition, while Type 2 diabetes is usually related to lifestyle factors. Gestational diabetes occurs during pregnancy.

4. Can diabetes be prevented?

Type 1 diabetes cannot be prevented, as it is caused by an autoimmune response. However, Type 2 diabetes can often be prevented or delayed through lifestyle modifications, such as maintaining a healthy diet, regular exercise, and weight management.

5. What is a diabetic diet?

A diabetic diet is a specialized eating plan designed to help individuals with diabetes manage their blood sugar levels. It focuses on balanced nutrition, portion control, and choosing foods with a lower glycemic index.

6. Can people with diabetes eat sweets and desserts?

Yes, people with diabetes can enjoy sweets and desserts in moderation as part of a balanced diet. It's essential to consider portion sizes and the total carbohydrate content to avoid blood sugar spikes.

7. What role does physical activity play in diabetes management?

Physical activity is crucial for diabetes management. Regular exercise helps improve insulin sensitivity, manage weight, and support overall health. It can also help regulate blood sugar levels.

8. Is diabetes a serious condition?

Yes, diabetes is a serious condition that requires ongoing management. Poorly controlled diabetes can lead to various complications affecting the heart, kidneys, nerves, and eyes.

9. Can diabetes lead to other health problems?

Yes, uncontrolled diabetes can lead to various health problems, including heart disease, kidney disease, nerve damage (neuropathy), and vision problems (retinopathy).

10. How often should blood sugar levels be checked?

The frequency of blood sugar monitoring varies depending on the type of diabetes, individual health, and treatment plan. People with diabetes may need to check their blood sugar levels multiple times a day or as recommended by their healthcare provider.

11. Can diabetes be cured?

Currently, there is no cure for diabetes. However, with proper management, individuals with diabetes can lead a healthy and fulfilling life while reducing the risk of complications.

Tips for Cooking

Cooking for a diabetic diet can be both enjoyable and beneficial for managing blood sugar levels and overall health. Here are some helpful tips for cooking in a diabetic-friendly way:

Focus on Balanced Meals: Aim to create balanced meals that include a variety of nutrients. Incorporate lean proteins, whole grains, healthy fats, and plenty of vegetables to promote stable blood sugar levels and overall well-being.

Choose Low-Glycemic Foods: Opt for foods with a low glycemic index (GI) to help prevent rapid spikes in blood sugar levels. Examples of low-GI foods include whole grains, legumes, non-starchy vegetables, and most fruits.

Limit Refined Carbohydrates and Sugars: Minimize or avoid highly processed and sugary foods. These can cause rapid increases in blood sugar levels and provide little nutritional value.

Use Healthy Cooking Methods: Opt for healthy cooking techniques such as baking, grilling, steaming, and sautéing instead of frying. These methods require less added fats and retain the natural flavors of the ingredients.

Watch Portion Sizes: Pay attention to portion sizes to prevent overeating, as consuming large amounts of any food, even healthy ones, can affect blood sugar levels.

Substitute Smartly: Make ingredient substitutions to reduce the carbohydrate or sugar content of a dish. For example, use whole wheat flour instead of white flour, or sweeten with natural alternatives like stevia or monk fruit.

Add Flavor with Herbs and Spices: Enhance the taste of your meals with herbs and spices instead of relying on excess salt or sugar. This will make your dishes more exciting without compromising on taste.

Choose Lean Proteins: Opt for lean sources of protein such as skinless poultry, fish, tofu, legumes, and beans. These provide essential nutrients without adding excessive saturated fat.

Control Sodium Intake: Be mindful of added sodium in recipes and use herbs, spices, and other seasonings to add flavor without relying on salt.

Incorporate Healthy Fats: Include sources of healthy fats like avocados, nuts, seeds, and olive oil in your cooking. These fats can help improve heart health and keep you feeling satisfied.

Plan Ahead: Plan your meals and snacks to ensure you have a well-balanced and diabetic-friendly menu throughout the week. This can help you make healthier choices and avoid impulsive decisions.

Stay Hydrated: Drink plenty of water throughout the day to stay hydrated and support optimal bodily functions.

Read Food Labels: When using packaged foods, read the nutritional labels to understand their carbohydrate, sugar, and fiber content. Choose products with lower sugar and higher fiber content.

Experiment with Recipes: Get creative in the kitchen and try new recipes that align with your dietary needs. Cooking at home allows you to have full control over the ingredients you use.

Consult a Dietitian: If you're unsure about meal planning or need personalized guidance, consider consulting a registered dietitian experienced in diabetes management.

By following these tips, you can create delicious and nutritious meals that support your diabetes management goals and promote overall health.

30 Days Diabetic Diet Meal Plan

DAYS	BREAKFAST	LUNCH	DINNER	SNACK/DESSERT
1	Tropical Steel Cut Oats P 14	Classic Oven-Roasted Carrots P 63	Raw Corn Salad with Black-Eyed Peas P 93	Peanut Butter Fudge Brownies P 101
2	Baked Oatmeal Cups P 14	Broccoli with Pine Nuts P 61	Cheeseburger Wedge Salad P 94	Cherry Almond Cobbler P 101
3	Peanut Butter Power Oats P 14	Mushroom "Bacon" Topper P 62	Crunchy Pecan Tuna Salad P 94	Superfood Brownie Bites P 102
4	Cherry, Chocolate, and Almond Shake P 14	Cheesy Broiled Tomatoes P 63	Rotisserie Chicken and Avocado Salad P 95	Chipotle Black Bean Brownies P 101
5	Cottage Cheese Almond Pancakes P 15	Blooming Onion P 63	Mediterranean Chicken Salad P 95	Baked Pumpkin Pudding P 103
6	Hash Browns P 16	Bacon-Wrapped Asparagus P 63	Three-Bean Salad with Black Bean Crumbles P 95	Oatmeal Chippers P 102
7	Breakfast Banana Barley P 15	Green Beans with Red Peppers P 62	Strawberry-Spinach Salad P 94	Blender Banana Snack Cake P 104
8	Egg-Stuffed Tomatoes P 14	Teriyaki Chickpeas P 63	Strawberry-Blueberry-Orange Salad P 94	Strawberry Cheesecake in a Jar P 103
9	Corn, Egg and Potato Bake P 15	Garlicky Cabbage and Collard Greens P 64	Mediterranean Pasta Salad with Goat Cheese P 93	Pineapple-Peanut Nice Cream P 104
10	Veggie-Stuffed Omelet P 15	Sautéed Mixed Vegetables P 64	Nutty Deconstructed Salad P 94	Blackberry Yogurt Ice Pops P 103
11	Crepe Cakes P 16	Green Bean and Radish Potato Salad P 62	Wild Rice Salad P 95	Berry Smoothie Pops P 103
12	Wild Mushroom Frittata P 17	Sweet-and-Sour Cabbage Slaw P 63	Herbed Spring Peas P 96	Avocado Chocolate Mousse P 105
13	Blueberry Coconut Breakfast Cookies P 17	Spicy Roasted Cauliflower with Lime P 64	Chicken Salad with Apricots P 96	Grilled Watermelon with Avocado Mousse P 105
14	Western Omelet P 16	Roasted Eggplant P 62	Herbed Tomato Salad P 93	Mango Nice Cream P 102
15	Easy Breakfast Chia Pudding P 16	Broiled Spinach P 64	Savory Skillet Corn Bread P 96	Mixed-Berry Cream Tart P 103
16	Rice Breakfast Bake P 17	Lean Green Avocado Mashed Potatoes P 61	Sofrito Steak Salad P 96	Banana Pineapple Freeze P 105
17	Whole-Grain Strawberry Pancakes P 16	Asparagus-Pepper Stir-Fry P 65	Sweet Beet Grain Bowl P 96	Dulce de Leche Fillo Cups P 105
18	Breakfast Panini P 18	Cauliflower Rice P 62	Apple-Bulgur Salad P 95	Banana Pudding P 104

DAYS	BREAKFAST	LUNCH	DINNER	SNACK/DESSERT
19	Veggie and Tofu Scramble P 19	Herb-Roasted Root Vegetables P 65	Crab and Rice Salad P 94	Vegetable Kabobs with Mustard Dip P 87
20	Very Cherry Overnight Oatmeal in a Jar P 19	Chinese Asparagus P 65	Garden-Fresh Greek Salad P 97	Peanut Butter Protein Bites P 90
21	Chorizo Mexican Breakfast Pizzas P 18	Sautéed Sweet Peppers P 65	Zucchini, Carrot, and Fennel Salad P 97	Spinach and Artichoke Dip P 86
22	Golden Potato Cakes P 19	Zucchini Noodles with Lime-Basil Pesto P 65	Three Bean and Basil Salad P 97	Lemon Artichokes P 86
23	Breakfast Sausage P 19	Fennel and Chickpeas P 66	Triple-Berry and Jicama Spinach Salad P 98	Hummus P 86
24	Fruity Avocado Smoothie P 17	Zucchini Ribbons with Tarragon P 97	Broccoli "Tabouli" P 98	Garlic Kale Chips P 88
25	Instant Pot Hard-Boiled Eggs P 15	Chipotle Twice-Baked Sweet Potatoes P 64	Carrot and Cashew Chicken Salad P 93	Cucumber Pâté P 89
26	Simple Buckwheat Porridge P 17	Parmesan Cauliflower Mash P 66	Couscous Salad P 98	Gruyere Apple Spread P 89
27	Sweet Potato Toasts P 19	Garlic Roasted Radishes P 67	Kidney Bean Salad P 97	7-Layer Dip P 88
28	Breakfast Meatballs P 20	Carrots Marsala P 67	Sunflower-Tuna-Cauliflower Salad P 98	Cocoa Coated Almonds P 88
29	Rice Breakfast Bake P 17	Ginger Broccoli P 66	Grilled Hearts of Romaine with Buttermilk Dressing P 99	Baked Scallops P 87
30	Maple Sausage Frittata P 20	Garlic Herb Radishes P 67	Broccoli Slaw Crab Salad P 99	Ground Turkey Lettuce Cups P 90

Chapter 3
Breakfasts

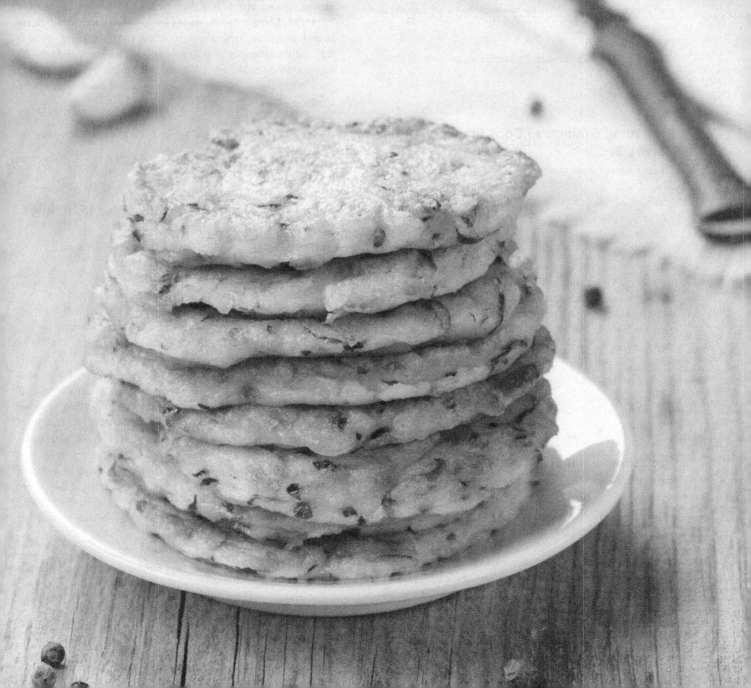

Tropical Steel Cut Oats

Prep time: 5 minutes | Cook time: 5 minutes | Serves 4

1 cup steel cut oats	1 (2-inch) vanilla bean, scraped (seeds and pod)
1 cup unsweetened almond milk	Ground cinnamon
2 cups coconut water or water	¼ cup chopped unsalted macadamia nuts
¾ cup frozen chopped peaches	
¾ cup frozen mango chunks	

1. In the electric pressure cooker, combine the oats, almond milk, coconut water, peaches, mango chunks, and vanilla bean seeds and pod. Stir well. 2. Close and lock the lid of the pressure cooker. Set the valve to sealing. 3. Cook on high pressure for 5 minutes. 4. When the cooking is complete, allow the pressure to release naturally for 10 minutes, then quick release any remaining pressure. Hit Cancel. 5. Once the pin drops, unlock and remove the lid. 6. Discard the vanilla bean pod and stir well. 7. Spoon the oats into 4 bowls. Top each serving with a sprinkle of cinnamon and 1 tablespoon of the macadamia nuts.

Per Serving:

calories: 127 | fat: 7g | protein: 2g | carbs: 14g | sugars: 8g | fiber: 3g | sodium: 167mg

Peanut Butter Power Oats

Prep time: 5 minutes | Cook time: 5 minutes | Serves 2

1½ cups unsweetened vanilla almond milk	butter
¾ cup rolled oats	2 tablespoons walnut pieces, divided (optional)
1 tablespoon chia seeds	¼ cup fresh berries, divided (optional)
2 tablespoons natural peanut	

1. In a small saucepan, bring the almond milk, oats, and chia seeds to a simmer. 2. Cover and cook, stirring frequently, until all of the milk is absorbed, and the chia seeds have gelled. 3. Add the peanut butter and stir until creamy. 4. Divide the oatmeal between two bowls. Top each serving with half of the walnuts and/or berries (if using).

Per Serving:

calories: 397 | fat: 12g | protein: 20g | carbs: 58g | sugars: 13g | fiber: 8g | sodium: 212mg

Cherry, Chocolate, and Almond Shake

Prep time: 5 minutes | Cook time: 0 minutes | Serves 2

10 ounces frozen cherries	2 tablespoons hemp seeds
2 tablespoons cocoa powder	8 ounces unsweetened almond milk
2 tablespoons almond butter	

1. Combine the cherries, cocoa, almond butter, hemp seeds, and almond milk in a blender and blend on high speed until smooth. Use a spatula to scrape down the sides as needed. Serve immediately.

Per Serving:

calories: 243 | fat: 16g | protein: 8g | carbs: 24g | sugars: 13g | fiber: 7g | sodium: 85mg

Baked Oatmeal Cups

Prep time: 5 minutes | Cook time: 20 minutes | Makes 15 cups

3 cups rolled oats	⅓ cup brown rice syrup
½ cup oat flour	⅓ cup raisins
3 tablespoons flax meal	2 tablespoons sugar-free nondairy chocolate chips (optional)
1 teaspoon cinnamon	
Rounded ⅛ teaspoon sea salt	
2 cups sliced overripe banana	

1. Line a muffin pan with 15 parchment cupcake liners. Preheat the oven to 350°F. 2. In a large mixing bowl, combine the oats, oat flour, flax meal, cinnamon, and salt. Stir to combine. Mash or puree the banana using a food processor or immersion blender. Add the banana, syrup, raisins, and chips (if using). Stir until thoroughly combined. Using a cookie scoop, place ¼ to ⅓ cup of the batter in each muffin cup. Use a spatula or your fingers to lightly pack in the mixture. (Dampen your fingers to make it easier.) Bake for 20 minutes. Remove and let cool in the pan for about 5 minutes, then transfer to a cooling rack. Enjoy warm or cooled. Store in an airtight container in the fridge.

Per Serving:

calorie: 133 | fat: 2g | protein: 3g | carbs: 27g | sugars: 7g | fiber: 3g | sodium: 37mg

Egg-Stuffed Tomatoes

Prep time: 20 minutes | Cook time: 15 minutes | Serves 4

1 teaspoon extra-virgin olive oil	¼ cup shredded low-fat Swiss cheese
4 large tomatoes	4 large eggs
¼ teaspoon sea salt, plus more for seasoning	1 tablespoon chopped fresh parsley
1 cup shredded kale	Freshly ground black pepper
2 tablespoons heavy (whipping) cream	

1. Preheat the oven to 375°F. 2. Lightly grease an 8-by-8-inch baking dish with the olive oil and set it aside. 3. Cut the tops off the tomatoes and carefully scoop out the insides, leaving the outer shells intact. 4. Sprinkle the insides of the tomatoes with ¼ teaspoon of salt and set them cut-side down on paper towels for 30 minutes. 5. Place the tomatoes in the baking dish, hollow-side up, and evenly divide the kale between them. 6. Divide the cream and cheese between the tomatoes. Carefully crack an egg on top of the cheese in each tomato. 7. Bake the tomatoes until the eggs are set, about 15 minutes. 8. Serve the stuffed tomatoes topped with parsley and seasoned lightly with salt and pepper.

Per Serving:

calories: 154 | fat: 9g | protein: 10g | carbs: 8g | sugars: 5g | fiber: 2g | sodium: 244mg

Breakfast Banana Barley

Prep time: 5 minutes | Cook time: 10 minutes | Serves 2

3 cups water

Pinch kosher salt

1½ cups quick barley, rinsed and drained

3 tablespoons natural peanut butter

1 banana, sliced

1. In a small saucepan, bring the water and salt to a boil over high heat. 2. Stir in the barley, cover, reduce the heat, and simmer for 10 minutes or until tender. 3. Remove the saucepan from the heat and add the peanut butter, stirring to blend. Adjust the salt as desired, and divide the mixture between two bowls. 4. Top with the sliced bananas and serve. 5. Store any leftovers in an airtight container in the refrigerator for up to 5 days.

Per Serving:

calories: 721 | fat: 11g | protein: 23g | carbs: 139g | sugars: 11g | fiber: 26g | sodium: 160mg

Corn, Egg and Potato Bake

Prep time: 20 minutes | Cook time: 1 hour | Serves 8

Monterey Jack cheese (6 ounces)

10 eggs or 2½ cups fat-free egg product

½ cup fat-free small-curd

cottage cheese

½ teaspoon dried oregano leaves

¼ teaspoon garlic powder

4 medium green onions, chopped (¼ cup)

1. Heat oven to 350°F. Spray 11x7-inch (2-quart) glass baking dish with cooking spray. In baking dish, layer potatoes, corn, bell peppers and 1 cup of the shredded cheese. 2. In medium bowl, beat eggs, cottage cheese, oregano and garlic powder with whisk until well blended. Slowly pour over potato mixture. Sprinkle with onions and remaining ½ cup shredded cheese. 3. Cover and bake 30 minutes. Uncover and bake about 30 minutes longer or until knife inserted in center comes out clean. Let stand 5 to 10 minutes before cutting.

Per Serving:

calories: 240 | fat: 11g | protein: 16g | carbs: 18g | sugars: 2g | fiber: 2g | sodium: 440mg

Veggie-Stuffed Omelet

Prep time: 15 minutes | Cook time: 10 minutes | Serves 1

1 teaspoon olive or canola oil

2 tablespoons chopped red bell pepper

1 tablespoon chopped onion

¼ cup sliced fresh mushrooms

1 cup loosely packed fresh baby spinach leaves, rinsed

½ cup fat-free egg product or 2 eggs, beaten

1 tablespoon water

Pinch salt

Pinch pepper

1 tablespoon shredded reduced-fat Cheddar cheese

1. In 8-inch nonstick skillet, heat oil over medium-high heat. Add bell pepper, onion and mushrooms to oil. Cook 2 minutes, stirring frequently, until onion is tender. Stir in spinach; continue cooking and stirring just until spinach wilts. Transfer vegetables from pan to small bowl. 2. In medium bowl, beat egg product, water, salt and pepper with fork or whisk until well mixed. Reheat same skillet over medium-high heat. Quickly pour egg mixture into pan. While sliding pan back and forth rapidly over heat, quickly stir with spatula to spread eggs continuously over bottom of pan as they thicken. Let stand over heat a few seconds to lightly brown bottom of omelet. Do not overcook; omelet will continue to cook after folding. 3. Place cooked vegetable mixture over half of omelet; top with cheese. With spatula, fold other half of omelet over vegetables. Gently slide out of pan onto plate. Serve immediately.

Per Serving:

calorie: 140 | fat: 5g | protein: 16g | carbs: 6g | sugars: 3g | fiber: 2g | sodium: 470mg

Cottage Cheese Almond Pancakes

Prep time: 10 minutes | Cook time: 20 minutes | Serves 4

2 cups low-fat cottage cheese

4 egg whites

2 eggs

1 tablespoon pure vanilla extract

1½ cups almond flour

Nonstick cooking spray

1. Place the cottage cheese, egg whites, eggs, and vanilla in a blender and pulse to combine. 2. Add the almond flour to the blender and blend until smooth. 3. Place a large nonstick skillet over medium heat and lightly coat it with cooking spray. 4. Spoon ¼ cup of batter per pancake, 4 at a time, into the skillet. Cook the pancakes until the bottoms are firm and golden, about 4 minutes. 5. Flip the pancakes over and cook the other side until they are cooked through, about 3 minutes. 6. Remove the pancakes to a plate and repeat with the remaining batter. 7. Serve with fresh fruit.

Per Serving:

calories: 441 | fat: 32g | protein: 30g | carbs: 9g | sugars: 3g | fiber: 5g | sodium: 528mg

Instant Pot Hard-Boiled Eggs

Prep time: 10 minutes | Cook time: 5 minutes | Serves 7

1 cup water

6 to 8 eggs

1. Pour the water into the inner pot. Place the eggs in a steamer basket or rack that came with pot. 2. Close the lid and secure to the locking position. Be sure the vent is turned to sealing. Set for 5 minutes on Manual at high pressure. (It takes about 5 minutes for pressure to build and then 5 minutes to cook.) 3. Let pressure naturally release for 5 minutes, then do quick pressure release. 4. Place hot eggs into cool water to halt cooking process. You can peel cooled eggs immediately or refrigerate unpeeled.

Per Serving:

calories: 72 | fat: 5g | protein: 6g | carbs: 0g | sugars: 0g | fiber: 0g | sodium: 71mg

Easy Breakfast Chia Pudding

Prep time: 5 minutes | Cook time: 0 minutes | Serves 4

4 cups unsweetened almond milk or skim milk	1 teaspoon ground cinnamon
¾ cup chia seeds	Pinch sea salt

1. Stir together the milk, chia seeds, cinnamon, and salt in a medium bowl. 2. Cover the bowl with plastic wrap and chill in the refrigerator until the pudding is thick, about 1 hour. 3. Sweeten with your favorite sweetener and fruit.

Per Serving:

calories: 129 | fat: 3g | protein: 10g | carbs: 16g | sugars: 12g | fiber: 3g | sodium: 131mg

Whole-Grain Strawberry Pancakes

Prep time: 30 minutes | Cook time: 10 minutes | Serves 7

1½ cups whole wheat flour	low-fat yogurt
3 tablespoons sugar	¾ cup water
1 teaspoon baking powder	3 tablespoons canola oil
½ teaspoon baking soda	1¾ cups sliced fresh strawberries
½ teaspoon salt	
3 eggs or ¾ cup fat-free egg product	1 container (6 ounces) strawberry low-fat yogurt
1 container (6 ounces) vanilla	

1. Heat griddle to 375°F or heat 12-inch skillet over medium heat. Grease with canola oil if necessary (or spray with cooking spray before heating). 2. In large bowl, mix flour, sugar, baking powder, baking soda and salt; set aside. In medium bowl, beat eggs, vanilla yogurt, water and oil with egg beater or whisk until well blended. Pour egg mixture all at once into flour mixture; stir until moistened. 3. For each pancake, pour slightly less than ¼ cup batter onto hot griddle. Cook pancakes 1 to 2 minutes or until bubbly on top, puffed and dry around edges. Turn; cook other sides 1 to 2 minutes or until golden brown. 4. Top each serving with ¼ cup sliced strawberries and 1 to 2 tablespoons strawberry yogurt.

Per Serving:

calories: 260 | fat: 9g | protein: 8g | carbs: 34g | sugars: 13g | fiber: 4g | sodium: 380mg

Hash Browns

Prep time: 5 minutes | Cook time: 10 minutes | Serves 4

2 large baking potatoes (about 10 ounces each), unpeeled	1 garlic clove, minced
2 tablespoons minced onion	½ teaspoon paprika
2 tablespoons minced red pepper	⅓ teaspoon salt
2 tablespoons minced green pepper	⅛ teaspoon freshly ground black pepper
	¼ teaspoon finely chopped fresh baby dill

1. With a hand grater or a food processor with grater attachment, shred each potato. In a large bowl, combine the potatoes with the remaining ingredients. 2. Coat a large skillet with cooking spray and place over medium heat until hot. 3. Pack the potato mixture firmly into the skillet; cook for 6 to 8 minutes or until the bottom is browned. Invert the potato patty onto a plate and return to the skillet, cooked side up. 4. Continue cooking over medium heat for another 6 to 8 minutes until the bottom is browned. Remove from heat and cut into 4 wedges.

Per Serving:

calories: 89 | fat: 0g | protein: 2g | carbs: 20g | sugars: 1g | fiber: 3g | sodium: 201mg

Crepe Cakes

Prep time: 5 minutes | Cook time: 20 minutes | Serves 4

Avocado oil cooking spray	4 large eggs
4 ounces reduced-fat plain cream cheese, softened	½ teaspoon vanilla extract
2 medium bananas	⅛ teaspoon salt

1. Heat a large skillet over low heat. Coat the cooking surface with cooking spray, and allow the pan to heat for another 2 to 3 minutes. 2. Meanwhile, in a medium bowl, mash the cream cheese and bananas together with a fork until combined. The bananas can be a little chunky. 3. Add the eggs, vanilla, and salt, and mix well. 4. For each cake, drop 2 tablespoons of the batter onto the warmed skillet and use the bottom of a large spoon or ladle to spread it thin. Let it cook for 7 to 9 minutes. 5. Flip the cake over and cook briefly, about 1 minute.

Per Serving:

calories: 183 | fat: 9g | protein: 9g | carbs: 16g | sugars: 9g | fiber: 2g | sodium: 251mg

Western Omelet

Prep time: 5 minutes | Cook time: 10 minutes | Serves 2

1½ teaspoons canola oil	pepper
¾ cup egg whites	2 tablespoons minced onion
¼ cup minced lean ham	⅛ teaspoon freshly ground black pepper
2 tablespoons minced green bell	

1. In a medium nonstick skillet over medium-low heat, heat the oil. 2. In a small mixing bowl, beat the egg whites slightly, and add the remaining ingredients along with a dash of salt, if desired. Pour the egg mixture into the heated skillet. 3. When the omelet begins to set, gently lift the edges of the omelet with a spatula, and tilt the skillet to allow the uncooked portion to flow underneath. Continue cooking until the eggs are firm. Then transfer to a serving platter.

Per Serving:

calories: 107 | fat: 4g | protein: 14g | carbs: 2g | sugars: 1g | fiber: 0g | sodium: 367mg

Wild Mushroom Frittata

Prep time: 10 minutes | Cook time: 15 minutes | Serves 4

8 large eggs	2 cups sliced wild mushrooms
½ cup skim milk	(cremini, oyster, shiitake,
¼ teaspoon ground nutmeg	portobello, etc.)
Sea salt	½ red onion, chopped
Freshly ground black pepper	1 teaspoon minced garlic
2 teaspoons extra-virgin olive oil	½ cup goat cheese, crumbled

1. Preheat the broiler. 2. In a medium bowl, whisk together the eggs, milk, and nutmeg until well combined. Season the egg mixture lightly with salt and pepper and set it aside. 3. Place an ovenproof skillet over medium heat and add the oil, coating the bottom completely by tilting the pan. 4. Sauté the mushrooms, onion, and garlic until translucent, about 7 minutes. 5. Pour the egg mixture into the skillet and cook until the bottom of the frittata is set, lifting the edges of the cooked egg to allow the uncooked egg to seep under. 6. Place the skillet under the broiler until the top is set, about 1 minute. 7. Sprinkle the goat cheese on the frittata and broil until the cheese is melted, about 1 minute more. 8. Remove from the oven. Cut into 4 wedges to serve.

Per Serving:

calories: 258 | fat: 17g | protein: 19g | carbs: 7g | sugars: 3g | fiber: 1g | sodium: 316mg

Rice Breakfast Bake

Prep time: 10 minutes | Cook time: 20 minutes | Serves 4

1¼ cups vanilla low-fat nondairy milk	(optional)
1 tablespoon ground chia seeds	1 teaspoon cinnamon
2½ cups cooked short-grain brown rice	½ teaspoon pure vanilla extract
	¼ teaspoon freshly grated nutmeg (optional)
2 cups sliced ripe (but not overripe) banana (2–2½ medium bananas)	Rounded ⅛ teaspoon sea salt
	2 tablespoons almond meal (or
1 cup chopped apple	1 tablespoon tigernut flour, for
2–3 tablespoons raisins	nut-free option)
	2 tablespoons coconut sugar

1. Preheat the oven to 400°F. 2. In a blender or food processor, combine the milk, ground chia, and 1 cup of the rice. Puree until fairly smooth. In a large bowl, combine the blended mixture, bananas, apple, raisins (if using), cinnamon, vanilla, nutmeg (if using), salt, and the remaining 1½ cups rice. Stir to fully combine. Transfer the mixture to a baking dish (8" x 8" or similar size). In a small bowl, combine the almond meal and sugar, and sprinkle it over the rice mixture. Cover with foil and bake for 15 minutes, then remove the foil and bake for another 5 minutes. Remove, let cool for 5 to 10 minutes, then serve.

Per Serving:

calorie: 334 | fat: 5g | protein: 7g | carbs: 69g | sugars: 22g | fiber: 7g | sodium: 145mg

Blueberry Coconut Breakfast Cookies

Prep time: 10 minutes | Cook time: 15 minutes | Serves 4

4 tablespoons unsalted butter, at room temperature	1 teaspoon vanilla extract
	⅔ cup coconut flour
2 medium bananas	¼ teaspoon salt
4 large eggs	1 cup fresh or frozen blueberries
½ cup unsweetened applesauce	

1. Preheat the oven to 375°F. 2. In a medium bowl, mash the butter and bananas together with a fork until combined. The bananas can be a little chunky. 3. Add the eggs, applesauce, and vanilla to the bananas and mix well. 4. Stir in the coconut flour and salt. 5. Gently fold in the blueberries. 6. Drop about 2 tablespoons of dough on a baking sheet for each cookie and flatten it a bit with the back of a spoon. Bake for about 13 minutes, or until firm to the touch.

Per Serving:

calories: 263 | fat: 15g | protein: 8g | carbs: 24g | sugars: 14g | fiber: 4g | sodium: 225mg

Fruity Avocado Smoothie

Prep time: 5 minutes | Cook time: 0 minutes | Serves 2

1 cup fresh spinach	½ cup blueberries
½ avocado, peeled, pitted, and diced	2 cups unsweetened almond milk
½ ripe banana, peeled	3 ice cubes

1. Put the spinach, avocado, banana, blueberries, almond milk, and ice cubes in a blender and blend until smooth. 2. Pour into two glasses and serve.

Per Serving:

calories: 178 | fat: 12g | protein: 3g | carbs: 18g | sugars: 8g | fiber: 6g | sodium: 186mg

Simple Buckwheat Porridge

Prep time: 5 minutes | Cook time: 40 minutes | Serves 4

2 cups raw buckwheat groats	Pinch sea salt
3 cups water	1 cup unsweetened almond milk

1. Put the buckwheat groats, water, and salt in a medium saucepan over medium-high heat. 2. Bring the mixture to a boil, then reduce the heat to low. 3. Cook until most of the water is absorbed, about 20 minutes. Stir in the milk and cook until very soft, about 15 minutes. 4. Serve the porridge with your favorite toppings such as chopped nuts, sliced banana, or fresh berries.

Per Serving:

calories: 314 | fat: 3g | protein: 10g | carbs: 67g | sugars: 5g | fiber: 9g | sodium: 52mg

Pumpkin–Peanut Butter Single-Serve Muffins

Prep time: 10 minutes | Cook time: 25 minutes | Serves 2

2 tablespoons powdered peanut butter	1 tablespoon dried cranberries
2 tablespoons coconut flour	½ cup water
2 tablespoons finely ground flaxseed	1 cup canned pumpkin
1 teaspoon pumpkin pie spice	2 large eggs
½ teaspoon baking powder	½ teaspoon vanilla extract
	Extra-virgin olive oil cooking spray

1. Preheat the oven to 350°F. 2. In a medium bowl, stir together the powdered peanut butter, coconut flour, flaxseed, pumpkin pie spice, baking powder, dried cranberries, and water. 3. In a separate medium bowl, whisk together the pumpkin and eggs until smooth. 4. Add the pumpkin mixture to the dry ingredients. Stir to combine. 5. Add the vanilla. Mix together well. 6. Spray 2 (8-ounce) ramekins with cooking spray. 7. Spoon half of the batter into each ramekin. 8. Place the ramekins on a baking and carefully transfer the sheet to the preheated oven. Bake for 25 minutes, or until a toothpick in the center comes out clean. Enjoy immediately!

Per Serving:

calories: 286 | fat: 16g | protein: 15g | carbs: 24g | sugars: 9g | fiber: 7g | sodium: 189mg

Stovetop Granola

Prep time: 10 minutes | Cook time: 10 minutes | Makes 4½ cups

1½ cups grains (rolled oats, rye flakes, or any flaked grain)	1¼ cups roasted, chopped nuts (almonds, walnuts, or pistachios)
¼ cup vegetable, grapeseed, or extra-virgin olive oil	¾ cup seeds (sunflower, pumpkin, sesame, hemp, ground chia, or ground flaxseed)
¼ cup honey or maple syrup	
1 tablespoon spice (cinnamon, chai spices, turmeric, ginger, or cloves)	½ cup dried fruit (golden raisins, apricots, raisins, dates, figs, or cranberries)
1 tablespoon citrus zest (orange, lemon, lime, or grapefruit) (optional)	Kosher salt

1. Heat a large dry skillet, preferably cast iron, over medium-high heat. Add the grains and cook, stirring frequently, until golden brown and toasty. Remove the grains from the skillet and transfer them to a small bowl. 2. Reduce the heat to medium, return the skillet to the heat, and add the vegetable oil, honey, and spice. Stir until thoroughly combined and bring to a simmer. 3. Once the mixture begins to bubble, reduce the heat to low and add the citrus zest (if using), toasted grains, nuts, seeds, and dried fruit. Stir and cook for another 2 minutes or until the granola is sticky and you can smell the spices. Adjust the seasonings as desired and add salt to taste. 4. Allow the granola to cool before storing it in an airtight container at room temperature for up to 6 months.

Per Serving:

½ cup: calories: 259 | fat: 13g | protein: 6g | carbs: 35g | sugars: 10g | fiber: 6g | sodium: 4mg

Breakfast Panini

Prep time: 10 minutes | Cook time: 10 minutes | Serves 2

2 eggs, beaten	2 slices tomato
½ teaspoon salt-free seasoning blend	2 thin slices onion
2 tablespoons chopped fresh chives	4 ultra-thin slices reduced-sodium deli ham
2 whole wheat thin bagels	2 thin slices reduced-fat Cheddar cheese

1. Spray 8-inch skillet with cooking spray; heat skillet over medium heat. In medium bowl, beat eggs, seasoning and chives with fork or whisk until well mixed. Pour into skillet. As eggs begin to set at bottom and side, gently lift cooked portions with spatula so that thin, uncooked portion can flow to bottom. Avoid constant stirring. Cook 3 to 4 minutes or until eggs are thickened throughout but still moist and creamy; remove from heat. 2. Meanwhile, heat closed contact grill or panini maker 5 minutes. 3. For each panini, divide cooked eggs evenly between bottom halves of bagels. Top each with 1 slice each tomato and onion, 2 ham slices, 1 cheese slice and top half of bagel. Transfer filled panini to heated grill. Close cover, pressing down lightly. Cook 2 to 3 minutes or until browned and cheese is melted. Serve immediately.

Per Serving:

1 Panini: calories: 260 | fat: 7g | protein: 15g | carbs: 32g | sugars: 5g | fiber: 2g | sodium: 410mg

Chorizo Mexican Breakfast Pizzas

Prep time: 15 minutes | Cook time: 15 minutes | Serves 4

6 ounces chorizo sausage, casing removed, crumbled, or 6 ounces bulk chorizo sausage	½ cup chopped tomatoes
	½ cup frozen whole-kernel corn, thawed
2 (10-inch) whole-grain lower-carb lavash flatbreads or tortillas	¼ cup reduced-fat shredded Cheddar cheese (1 ounce)
¼ cup chunky-style salsa	1 tablespoon chopped fresh cilantro
½ cup black beans with cumin and chili spices (from 15-ounce can)	2 teaspoons crumbed cotija (white Mexican) cheese

1. Heat oven to 425°F. In 8-inch skillet, cook sausage over medium heat 4 to 5 minutes or until brown; drain. 2. On 1 large or 2 small cookie sheets, place flatbreads. Spread each with 2 tablespoons salsa. Top each with half the chorizo, beans, tomatoes, corn and Cheddar cheese. 3. Bake about 8 minutes or until cheese is melted. Sprinkle each with half the cilantro and cotija cheese; cut into wedges. Serve immediately.

Per Serving:

calories: 330 | fat: 2g | protein: 20g | carbs: 19g | sugars: 2g | fiber: 6g | sodium: 1030mg

Veggie and Tofu Scramble

Prep time: 5 minutes | Cook time: 10 minutes | Serves 2

1 pound firm- or extra-firm tofu	2 garlic cloves, minced
1 teaspoon dry mustard	1 bunch spinach, rinsed and
1 teaspoon ground cumin	chopped
1 tablespoon extra-virgin olive	½ teaspoon low-sodium soy
oil	sauce
2 medium tomatoes, diced	1 teaspoon freshly squeezed
1 medium zucchini, chopped	lemon juice
¾ cup sliced fresh mushrooms	Freshly ground black pepper

1. In a colander, drain the tofu. 2. In a medium bowl, crumble the drained tofu. 3. Add the mustard and cumin. Toss until well mixed. 4. In a nonstick skillet set over medium-high heat, heat the olive oil. 5. Add the tomatoes, zucchini, mushrooms, and garlic. Sauté for 2 to 3 minutes. Reduce the heat to medium-low. 6. Add the spinach, tofu, soy sauce, and lemon juice. 7. Cover and cook for 5 to 7 minutes, stirring occasionally. 8. Season with pepper and serve immediately.

Per Serving:

calories: 293 | fat: 16g | protein: 23g | carbs: 21g | sugars: 9g | fiber: 7g | sodium: 239mg

Very Cherry Overnight Oatmeal in a Jar

Prep time: 30 minutes | Cook time: 0 minutes | Serves 2

½ cup uncooked old-fashioned	1 teaspoon liquid stevia
rolled oats	1 teaspoon cinnamon
½ cup nonfat milk	½ teaspoon vanilla extract
½ cup plain nonfat Greek yogurt	½ cup frozen cherries, divided
2 tablespoons chia seeds	

1. In a small bowl, mix together the oats, milk, yogurt, chia seeds, stevia, cinnamon, and vanilla. 2. Evenly divide the oat mixture between 2 mason jars or individual containers. Cover tightly and shake until well combined. 3. To each jar, stir in ¼ cup of cherries. 4. Seal the containers and refrigerate overnight. 5. The next day, enjoy chilled or heated.

Per Serving:

calories: 247 | fat: 4g | protein: 13g | carbs: 41g | sugars: 11g | fiber: 7g | sodium: 81mg

Golden Potato Cakes

Prep time: 10 minutes | Cook time: 25 minutes | Serves 4

½ pound russet potatoes, peeled, shredded, rinsed, and patted dry	Sea salt
¼ sweet onion, chopped	Freshly ground black pepper
1 teaspoon extra-virgin olive oil	Nonstick cooking spray
1 teaspoon chopped fresh thyme	1 cup unsweetened applesauce

1. Place the potatoes, onion, oil, and thyme in a large bowl and stir to mix well. 2. Season the potato mixture generously with salt and pepper. 3. Place a large skillet over medium heat and lightly coat it with cooking spray. 4. Scoop about ¼ cup of potato mixture per cake into the skillet and press down with a spatula, about 4 cakes per batch. 5. Cook until the bottoms are golden brown and firm, about 5 to 7 minutes, then flip the cake over. Cook the other side until it is golden brown and the cake is completely cooked through, about 5 minutes more. 6. Remove the cakes to a plate and repeat with the remaining mixture. 7. Serve with the applesauce.

Per Serving:

calories: 88 | fat: 1g | protein: 1g | carbs: 19g | sugars: 7g | fiber: 2g | sodium: 6mg

Breakfast Sausage

Prep time: 15 minutes | Cook time: 15 minutes | Serves 10

½ red bell pepper, minced	1 pound ground turkey
½ orange bell pepper, minced	¼ teaspoon smoked paprika
½ jalapeño pepper, minced	¼ teaspoon ground cumin
1 cup roughly chopped tomatoes	1 tablespoon Worcestershire
1 garlic clove, minced	sauce
1 pound ground chicken	

1. Preheat the oven to 350°F. 2. In a large bowl, combine the red bell pepper, orange bell pepper, jalapeño pepper, tomatoes, garlic, chicken, turkey, paprika, cumin, and Worcestershire sauce. Gently fold together until well mixed. 3. With clean hands, take about ⅓-cup portions, and shape into balls about the size of a golf ball. 4. Gently press the balls into flat disks, and place on a rimmed baking sheet in a single layer at least 1 inch apart. Repeat with the remaining meat. You should have 10 patties. 5. Transfer the baking sheet to the oven and cook for 5 to 7 minutes. 6. Flip the patties and cook for 5 to 7 minutes, or until the juices run clear. 7. Serve.

Per Serving:

calories: 110 | fat: 2g | protein: 21g | carbs: 2g | sugars: 1g | fiber: 1g | sodium: 64mg

Sweet Potato Toasts

Prep time: 10 minutes | Cook time: 2 minutes | Serves 1

2 slices sprouted grain bread	Freshly ground black pepper
½ cup mashed cooked sweet	(optional)
potato, peel removed	2 tablespoons cubed avocado or
½ to 1 teaspoon lemon juice	1 tablespoon sliced black olives
A couple pinches of sea salt	

1. Toast the bread. In a small bowl, mash the sweet potato with the lemon juice (adjusting to taste), salt, and pepper (if using). Distribute the mashed sweet potato between the slices of toast, and top with either the cubed avocado or the black olives. Serve!

Per Serving:

calorie: 312 | fat: 5g | protein: 8g | carbs: 59g | sugars: 11g | fiber: 8g | sodium: 1018mg

Breakfast Meatballs

Prep time: 10 minutes | Cook time: 15 minutes | Makes 18 meatballs

1 pound (454 g) ground pork breakfast sausage	cheese
½ teaspoon salt	1 ounce (28 g) cream cheese, softened
¼ teaspoon ground black pepper	1 large egg, whisked
½ cup shredded sharp Cheddar	

1. Combine all ingredients in a large bowl. Form mixture into eighteen 1-inch meatballs. 2. Place meatballs into ungreased air fryer basket. Adjust the temperature to 400ºF (204ºC) and air fry for 15 minutes, shaking basket three times during cooking. Meatballs will be browned on the outside and have an internal temperature of at least 145ºF (63ºC) when completely cooked. Serve warm.

Per Serving:

1 meatball: calories: 106 | fat: 9g | protein: 5g | carbs: 0g | sugars: 0g | fiber: 0g | sodium: 284mg

Maple Sausage Frittata

Prep time: 10 minutes | Cook time: 15 minutes | Serves 4

Avocado oil cooking spray	¾ cup half-and-half
1 cup roughly chopped portobello mushrooms	¼ cup unsweetened almond milk
1 medium green bell pepper, diced	6 links maple-flavored chicken or turkey breakfast sausage, cut
1 medium red bell pepper, diced	into ¼-inch pieces
8 large eggs	

1. Preheat the oven to 375ºF. 2. Heat a large, oven-safe skillet over medium-low heat. When hot, coat the cooking surface with cooking spray. 3. Heat the mushrooms, green bell pepper, and red bell pepper in the skillet. Cook for 5 minutes. 4. Meanwhile, in a medium bowl, whisk the eggs, half-and-half, and almond milk. 5. Add the sausage to the skillet and cook for 2 minutes. 6. Pour the egg mixture into the skillet, then transfer the skillet from the stove to the oven, and bake for 15 minutes, or until the middle is firm and spongy.

Per Serving:

calories: 245 | fat: 14g | protein: 18g | carbs: 10g | sugars: 6g | fiber: 2g | sodium: 334mg

Breakfast Hash

Prep time: 10 minutes | Cook time: 30 minutes | Serves 6

Oil, for spraying	2 tablespoons olive oil
3 medium russet potatoes, diced	2 teaspoons granulated garlic
½ yellow onion, diced	1 teaspoon salt
1 green bell pepper, seeded and diced	½ teaspoon freshly ground black pepper

1. Line the air fryer basket with parchment and spray lightly with oil. 2. In a large bowl, mix together the potatoes, onion, bell pepper,

and olive oil. 3. Add the garlic, salt, and black pepper and stir until evenly coated. 4. Transfer the mixture to the prepared basket. 5. Air fry at 400ºF (204ºC) for 20 to 30 minutes, shaking or stirring every 10 minutes, until browned and crispy. If you spray the potatoes with a little oil each time you stir, they will get even crispier.

Per Serving:

calorie: 124 | fat: 4g | protein: 2g | carbs: 21g | sugars: 2g | fiber: 2g | sodium: 390mg

Spicy Tomato Smoothie

Prep time: 5 minutes | Cook time: 0 minutes | Serves 2

1 cup tomato juice	Juice of 1 lemon
2 tomatoes, diced	1 teaspoon hot sauce
¼ English cucumber	4 ice cubes

1. Put the tomato juice, tomatoes, cucumber, lemon juice, hot sauce, and ice cubes in a blender and blend until smooth. 2. Pour into two glasses and serve.

Per Serving:

calories: 51 | fat: 1g | protein: 2g | carbs: 11g | sugars: 7g | fiber: 2g | sodium: 34mg

Lentil, Squash, and Tomato Omelet

Prep time: 5 minutes | Cook time: 45 minutes | Serves 2

1 cup water	chopped
⅓ cup dried lentils, picked over, rinsed, and drained	1 garlic clove, chopped
Extra-virgin olive oil cooking spray	2 tablespoons chopped fresh chives
1 medium zucchini, thinly sliced	2 large eggs
½ cup grape tomatoes, coarsely	2 tablespoons nonfat milk

1. Preheat the oven to 350°F. 2. In a small saucepan set over high heat, heat the water until it boils. 3. Add the lentils. Reduce the heat to low. Simmer for about 15 minutes, or until most of the liquid has been absorbed. In a colander, drain and set aside. 4. Lightly coat an 8- or 9-inch nonstick skillet with cooking spray. Place the skillet over medium-high heat. 5. Add the zucchini, tomatoes, garlic, and chives. Sauté for 5 to 10 minutes, stirring frequently, or until soft. 6. Add the lentils to the skillet. 7. In a medium bowl, beat together the eggs and milk with a fork. 8. Lightly coat a small casserole or baking dish with cooking spray. 9. In the bottom of the prepared dish, spread the vegetable mixture. 10. Pour the egg mixture over. Use a fork to distribute evenly. 11. Place the dish in the preheated oven. Bake for 15 to 20 minutes, or until the dish is set in the middle. 12. Slice in half and enjoy!

Per Serving:

calories: 209 | fat: 6g | protein: 16g | carbs: 25g | sugars: 4g | fiber: 5g | sodium: 90mg

Chocolate-Zucchini Muffins

Prep time: 15 minutes | Cook time: 20 minutes | Serves 12

1½ cups grated zucchini	1 teaspoon vanilla extract
1½ cups rolled oats	¼ cup coconut oil, melted
1 teaspoon ground cinnamon	½ cup unsweetened applesauce
2 teaspoons baking powder	¼ cup honey
¼ teaspoon salt	¼ cup dark chocolate chips
1 large egg	

1. Preheat the oven to 350°F. Grease the cups of a 12-cup muffin tin or line with paper baking liners. Set aside. 2. Place the zucchini in a colander over the sink to drain. 3. In a blender jar, process the oats until they resemble flour. Transfer to a medium mixing bowl and add the cinnamon, baking powder, and salt. Mix well. 4. In another large mixing bowl, combine the egg, vanilla, coconut oil, applesauce, and honey. Stir to combine. 5. Press the zucchini into the colander, draining any liquids, and add to the wet mixture. 6. Stir the dry mixture into the wet mixture, and mix until no dry spots remain. Fold in the chocolate chips. 7. Transfer the batter to the muffin tin, filling each cup a little over halfway. Cook for 16 to 18 minutes until the muffins are lightly browned and a toothpick inserted in the center comes out clean. 8. Store in an airtight container, refrigerated, for up to 5 days.

Per Serving:

calories: 121 | fat: 7g | protein: 2g | carbs: 16g | sugars: 7g | fiber: 2g | sodium: 106mg

Easy Buckwheat Crêpes

Prep time: 5 minutes | Cook time: 15 minutes | Makes 12 crêpes

1 cup buckwheat flour	oil
1¾ cups milk	½ tablespoon ground flaxseed
⅛ teaspoon kosher salt	(optional)
1 tablespoon extra-virgin olive	

1. Combine the buckwheat flour, milk, salt, extra-virgin olive oil, and flaxseed (if using), in a bowl and whisk thoroughly, or in a blender and pulse until well combined. 2. Heat a nonstick medium skillet over medium heat. Once it's hot, add a ¼ cup of batter to the skillet, spreading it out evenly. Cook until bubbles appear and the edges crisp like a pancake, 1 to 3 minutes, then flip and cook for another 2 minutes. 3. Repeat until all the batter is used up, and the crêpes are cooked. Layer parchment paper or tea towels between the crêpes to keep them from sticking to one another while also keeping them warm until you're ready to eat. 4. Serve with the desired fillings. 5. Store any leftovers in an airtight container in the refrigerator for up to 3 days.

Per Serving:

1 crêpes: calories: 56 | fat: 2g | protein: 2g | carbs: 9g | sugars: 2g | fiber: 1g | sodium: 46mg

Baked French Toast with Raspberry Sauce

Prep time: 5 minutes | Cook time: 30 minutes | Serves 4

1 cup egg substitute	2 cups frozen or fresh
⅔ cup fat-free milk	raspberries
1 teaspoon cinnamon	1 tablespoon orange juice
½ teaspoon nutmeg	1 teaspoon vanilla extract
8 slices whole-wheat bread	2 teaspoons cornstarch

1. In a medium bowl, beat together the egg substitute, milk, cinnamon, and nutmeg. 2. In a casserole dish, lay the bread slices side by side. Pour on the egg-milk mixture, cover, and refrigerate overnight. 3. The next day, bake the French toast at 350 degrees for about 30 minutes until golden brown and slightly puffed. 4. To make the raspberry sauce, puree the raspberries in a blender. Strain to remove the seeds. 5. In a small saucepan, combine the pureed berries with the orange juice, vanilla, and cornstarch. Bring to a boil and cook for 1 minute until the mixture is thickened. Serve over French toast.

Per Serving:

calories: 250 | fat: 3g | protein: 16g | carbs: 40g | sugars: 9g | fiber: 8g | sodium: 433mg

BLT Breakfast Wrap

Prep time: 5 minutes | Cook time: 10 minutes | Serves 4

8 ounces (227 g) reduced-sodium bacon	4 Roma tomatoes, sliced
8 tablespoons mayonnaise	Salt and freshly ground black pepper, to taste
8 large romaine lettuce leaves	

1. Arrange the bacon in a single layer in the air fryer basket. (It's OK if the bacon sits a bit on the sides.) Set the air fryer to 350°F (177°C) and air fry for 10 minutes. Check for crispiness and air fry for 2 to 3 minutes longer if needed. Cook in batches, if necessary, and drain the grease in between batches. 2. Spread 1 tablespoon of mayonnaise on each of the lettuce leaves and top with the tomatoes and cooked bacon. Season to taste with salt and freshly ground black pepper. Roll the lettuce leaves as you would a burrito, securing with a toothpick if desired.

Per Serving:

calorie: 465 | fat: 41g | protein: 14g | carbs: 8g | sugars: 4g | fiber: 3g | sodium: 861mg

Sausage, Sweet Potato, and Kale Hash

Prep time: 10 minutes | Cook time: 15 minutes | Serves 4

Avocado oil cooking spray

1⅓ cups peeled and diced sweet potatoes

8 cups roughly chopped kale, stemmed and loosely packed (about 2 bunches)

4 links chicken or turkey breakfast sausage

4 large eggs

4 lemon wedges

1. Heat a large skillet over medium heat. When hot, coat the cooking surface with cooking spray. Cook the sweet potatoes for 4 minutes, stirring once halfway through. 2. Reduce the heat to medium-low and move the potatoes to one side of the skillet. Arrange the kale and sausage in a single layer. Cover and cook for 3 minutes. 3. Stir the vegetables and sausage together, then push them to one side of the skillet to create space for the eggs. Add the eggs and cook them to your liking. Cover the skillet and cook for 3 minutes. 4. Divide the sausage and vegetables into four equal portions and top with an egg and a squeeze of lemon.

Per Serving:

calories: 160 | fat: 8g | protein: 11g | carbs: 13g | sugars: 3g | fiber: 3g | sodium: 197mg

Triple-Berry Oatmeal Muesli

Prep time: 25 minutes | Cook time: 18 to 20 minutes | Serves 6

2¾ cups old-fashioned oats or rolled barley

½ cup sliced almonds

2 containers (6 ounces each) banana crème or French vanilla fat-free yogurt

1½ cups milk

¼ cup ground flaxseed or flaxseed meal

½ cup fresh blueberries

½ cup fresh raspberries

½ cup sliced fresh strawberries

1. Heat oven to 350°F. On cookie sheet, spread oats and almonds. Bake 18 to 20 minutes, stirring occasionally, until light golden brown; cool 15 minutes. 2. In large bowl, mix yogurt and milk until well blended. Stir in oats, almonds and flaxseed. Divide muesli evenly among 6 bowls. Top each serving with berries.

Per Serving:

calorie: 320 | fat: 10g | protein: 11g | carbs: 46g | sugars: 15g | fiber: 11g | sodium: 65mg

Chapter 4
Beans and Grains

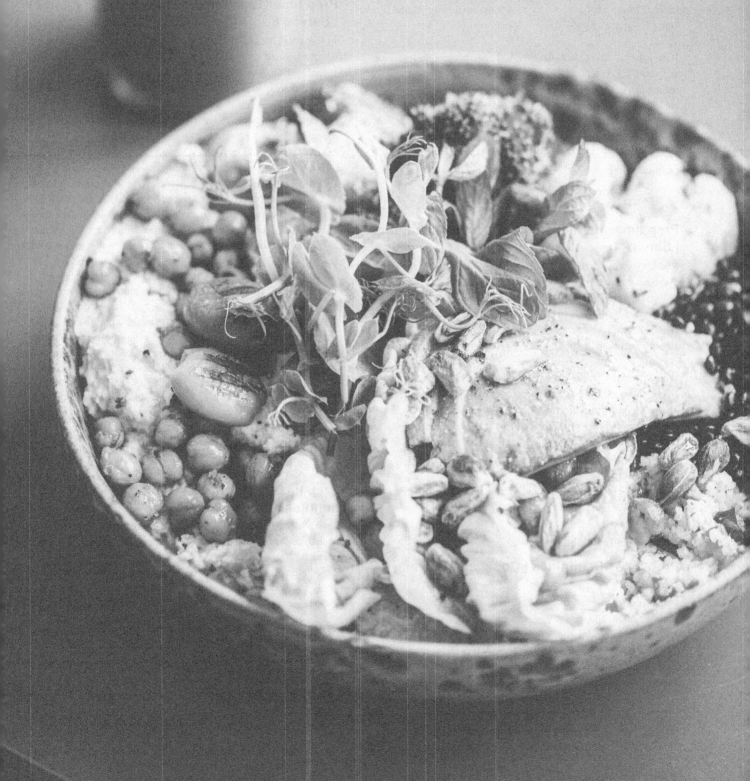

Colorful Rice Casserole

Prep time: 5 minutes | Cook time: 20 minutes | Serves 12

1 tablespoon extra-virgin olive oil	added chopped tomatoes, undrained
1½ pounds zucchini, thinly sliced	¼ cup chopped parsley
¾ cup chopped scallions	1 teaspoon oregano
2 cups corn kernels (frozen or fresh; if frozen, defrost)	3 cups cooked brown (or white) rice
One 14½-ounce can no-salt-	⅛ teaspoon freshly ground black pepper

1. In a large skillet, heat the oil. Add the zucchini and scallions, and sauté for 5 minutes. 2. Add the remaining ingredients, cover, reduce heat, and simmer for 10–15 minutes or until the vegetables are heated through. Season with salt, if desired, and pepper. Transfer to a bowl, and serve.

Per Serving:

calorie: 109 | fat: 2g | protein: 3g | carbs: 21g | sugars: 4g | fiber: 3g | sodium: 14mg

Beet Greens and Black Beans

Prep time: 10 minutes | Cook time: 20 minutes | Serves 4

1 tablespoon unsalted non-hydrogenated plant-based butter	ribbons
½ Vidalia onion, thinly sliced	1 bunch dandelion greens, cut into ribbons
½ cup store-bought low-sodium vegetable broth	1 (15-ounce) can no-salt-added black beans
1 bunch beet greens, cut into	Freshly ground black pepper

1. In a medium skillet, melt the butter over low heat. 2. Add the onion, and sauté for 3 to 5 minutes, or until the onion is translucent. 3. Add the broth and greens. Cover the skillet and cook for 7 to 10 minutes, or until the greens are wilted. 4. Add the black beans and cook for 3 to 5 minutes, or until the beans are tender. Season with black pepper.

Per Serving:

calorie: 153 | fat: 3g | protein: 9g | carbs: 25g | sugars: 2g | fiber: 11g | sodium: 312mg

Bulgur and Eggplant Pilaf

Prep time: 10 minutes | Cook time: 1 hour | Serves 4

1 tablespoon extra-virgin olive oil	broth
½ sweet onion, chopped	1 cup diced tomato
2 teaspoons minced garlic	Sea salt
1 cup chopped eggplant	Freshly ground black pepper
1½ cups bulgur	2 tablespoons chopped fresh basil
4 cups low-sodium chicken	

1. Place a large saucepan over medium-high heat. Add the oil and sauté the onion and garlic until softened and translucent, about 3 minutes. 2. Stir in the eggplant and sauté 4 minutes to soften. 3. Stir in the bulgur, broth, and tomatoes. Bring the mixture to a boil. 4. Reduce the heat to low, cover, and simmer until the water has been absorbed, about 50 minutes. 5. Season the pilaf with salt and pepper. 6. Garnish with the basil, and serve.

Per Serving:

calorie: 372 | fat: 7g | protein: 15g | carbs: 65g | sugars: 8g | fiber: 18g | sodium: 77mg

Baked Vegetable Macaroni Pie

Prep time: 15 minutes | Cook time: 35 minutes | Serves 6

1 (16-ounce) package whole-wheat macaroni	1 cup fat-free milk
1 small yellow onion, chopped	2 cups grated reduced-fat sharp Cheddar cheese
2 garlic cloves, minced	2 large zucchini, finely grated and squeezed dry
2 celery stalks, thinly sliced	2 roasted red peppers, chopped into ¼-inch pieces
¼ teaspoon freshly ground black pepper	
2 tablespoons chickpea flour	

1. Preheat the oven to 350°F. 2. Bring a large pot of water to a boil. 3. Add the macaroni and cook for 2 to 5 minutes, or until al dente. 4. Drain the macaroni, reserving 1 cup of the pasta water for the cheese sauce. Rinse under cold running water, and transfer to a large bowl. 5. In a large cast iron skillet, warm the pasta water over medium heat. 6. Add the onion, garlic, celery, and pepper. Cook for 3 to 5 minutes, or until the onion is translucent. 7. Add the chickpea flour slowly, mixing often. 8. Stir in the milk and cheese until a thick liquid is formed. It should be about the consistency of a smoothie. 9. Add the pasta to the cheese mixture along with the zucchini and red peppers. Mix thoroughly so the ingredients are evenly dispersed. 10. Cover the skillet tightly with aluminum foil, transfer to the oven, and bake for 15 to 20 minutes, or until the cheese is well melted. 11. Uncover and bake for 5 minutes, or until golden brown.

Per Serving:

calorie: 382 | fat: 4g | protein: 24g | carbs: 67g | sugars: 6g | fiber: 8g | sodium: 373mg

Sage and Garlic Vegetable Bake

Prep time: 30 minutes | Cook time: 1 hour 15 minutes | Serves 6

1 medium butternut squash, peeled, cut into 1-inch pieces (3 cups)	1 medium onion, coarsely chopped (½ cup)
2 medium parsnips, peeled, cut into 1-inch pieces (2 cups)	½ cup uncooked quick-cooking barley
2 cans (14½ ounces each) stewed tomatoes, undrained	½ cup water
2 cups frozen cut green beans	1 teaspoon dried sage leaves
	½ teaspoon seasoned salt
	2 cloves garlic, finely chopped

1. Heat oven to 375°F. In ungreased 3-quart casserole, mix all ingredients, breaking up large pieces of tomatoes. 2. Cover; bake 1 hour to 1 hour 15 minutes or until vegetables and barley are tender.

Per Serving:

calorie: 170 | fat: 0g | protein: 4g | carbs: 37g | sugars: 9g | fiber: 8g | sodium: 410mg

Barley Squash Risotto

Prep time: 10 minutes | Cook time: 15 minutes | Serves 6

1 teaspoon extra-virgin olive oil	cut into ½-inch cubes
½ sweet onion, finely chopped	2 tablespoons chopped
1 teaspoon minced garlic	pistachios
2 cups cooked barley	1 tablespoon chopped fresh
2 cups chopped kale	thyme
2 cups cooked butternut squash,	Sea salt

1. Place a large skillet over medium heat and add the oil. 2. Sauté the onion and garlic until softened and translucent, about 3 minutes. 3. Add the barley and kale, and stir until the grains are heated through and the greens are wilted, about 7 minutes. 4. Stir in the squash, pistachios, and thyme. 5. Cook until the dish is hot, about 4 minutes, and season with salt.

Per Serving:

calorie: 158 | fat: 3g | protein: 4g | carbs: 31g | sugars: 3g | fiber: 7g | sodium: 77mg

Green Lentils with Olives and Summer Vegetables

Prep time: 15 minutes | Cook time: 0 minutes | Serves 4

3 tablespoons extra-virgin olive oil	2 (15 ounces) cans sodium-free green lentils, rinsed and drained
2 tablespoons balsamic vinegar	½ English cucumber, diced
2 teaspoons chopped fresh basil	2 tomatoes, diced
1 teaspoon minced garlic	½ cup halved Kalamata olives
Sea salt	¼ cup chopped fresh chives
Freshly ground black pepper	2 tablespoons pine nuts

1. Whisk together the olive oil, vinegar, basil, and garlic in a medium bowl. Season with salt and pepper. 2. Stir in the lentils, cucumber, tomatoes, olives, and chives. 3. Top with the pine nuts, and serve.

Per Serving:

calorie: 476 | fat: 29g | protein: 17g | carbs: 42g | sugars: 5g | fiber: 16g | sodium: 404mg

Edamame-Tabbouleh Salad

Prep time: 20 minutes | Cook time: 10 minutes | Serves 6

Salad	2 medium tomatoes, seeded,
1 package (5.8 ounces) roasted	chopped (1½ cups)
garlic and olive oil couscous	1 small cucumber, peeled,
mix	chopped (1 cup)
1¼ cups water	¼ cup chopped fresh parsley
1 teaspoon olive or canola oil	Dressing
1 bag (10 ounces) refrigerated	1 teaspoon grated lemon peel
fully cooked ready-to-eat shelled	2 tablespoons lemon juice
edamame (green soybeans)	1 teaspoon olive or canola oil

1. Make couscous mix as directed on package, using the water and oil. 2. In large bowl, mix couscous and remaining salad ingredients. In small bowl, mix dressing ingredients. Pour dressing over salad; mix well. Serve immediately, or cover and refrigerate until serving time.

Per Serving:

calorie: 200 | fat: 5g | protein: 10g | carbs: 28g | sugars: 3g | fiber: 4g | sodium: 270mg

Green Chickpea Falafel

Prep time: 10 minutes | Cook time: 11 to 12 minutes | Serves 4

1 bag (14 ounces) green chickpeas, thawed (about 3½ cups)	2 medium-large cloves garlic
	2 teaspoons ground cumin
	½ teaspoon turmeric
½ cup fresh flat-leaf parsley leaves	1 teaspoon ground coriander
	1 teaspoon sea salt
½ cup fresh cilantro leaves	¼ to ½ teaspoon crushed red-pepper flakes
1½ tablespoons freshly squeezed lemon juice	1 cup rolled oats

1. In a food processor, combine the chickpeas, parsley, cilantro, lemon juice, garlic, cumin, turmeric, coriander, salt, and red-pepper flakes. (Use ¼ teaspoon if you like it mild and ½ teaspoon if you like it spicier.) Process until the mixture breaks down and begins to smooth out. Add the oats and pulse a few times to work them in. Refrigerate for 30 minutes, if possible. 2. Preheat the oven to 400°F. Line a baking sheet with parchment paper. 3. Use a cookie scoop to take small scoops of the mixture, 1 to 1½ tablespoons each. Place falafel balls on the prepared baking sheet. Bake for 11 to 12 minutes, until the falafel balls begin to firm (they will still be tender inside) and turn golden in spots.

Per Serving:

calorie: 253 | fat: 4g | protein: 12g | carbs: 43g | sugars: 5g | fiber: 10g | sodium: 601mg

Hoppin' John

Prep time: 15 minutes | Cook time: 50 minutes | Serves 12

1 tablespoon canola oil	2 cups brown rice, rinsed
2 celery stalks, thinly sliced	5 cups store-bought low-sodium
1 small yellow onion, chopped	vegetable broth, divided
1 medium green bell pepper,	2 bay leaves
chopped	1 teaspoon smoked paprika
1 tablespoon tomato paste	1 teaspoon Creole seasoning
2 garlic cloves, minced	1¼ cups frozen black-eyed peas

1. In a Dutch oven, heat the canola oil over medium heat. 2. Add the celery, onion, bell pepper, tomato paste, and garlic and cook, stirring often, for 3 to 5 minutes, or until the vegetables are softened. 3. Add the rice, 4 cups of broth, bay leaves, paprika, and Creole seasoning. 4. Reduce the heat to low, cover, and cook for 30 minutes, or until the rice is tender. 5. Add the black-eyed peas and remaining 1 cup of broth. Mix well, cover, and cook for 12 minutes, or until the peas soften. Discard the bay leaves. 6. Enjoy.

Per Serving:

calorie: 155 | fat: 2g | protein: 4g | carbs: 30g | sugars: 1g | fiber: 2g | sodium: 24mg

Sweet Potato Fennel Bake

Prep time: 15 minutes | Cook time: 45 minutes | Serves 4

1 teaspoon butter	to taste
1 fennel bulb, trimmed and thinly sliced	½ teaspoon ground cinnamon
2 sweet potatoes, peeled and thinly sliced	¼ teaspoon ground nutmeg
Freshly ground black pepper,	1 cup low-sodium vegetable broth

1. Preheat the oven to 375°F. 2. Lightly butter a 9-by-11-inch baking dish. 3. Arrange half the fennel in the bottom of the dish and top with half the sweet potatoes. 4. Season the potatoes with black pepper. Sprinkle half the cinnamon and nutmeg on the potatoes. 5. Repeat the layering to use up all the fennel, sweet potatoes, cinnamon, and nutmeg. 6. Pour in the vegetable broth and cover the dish with aluminum foil. 7. Bake until the vegetables are very tender, about 45 minutes. 8. Serve immediately.

Per Serving:

calorie: 118 | fat: 1g | protein: 2g | carbs: 28g | sugars: 7g | fiber: 5g | sodium: 127mg

Southwestern Quinoa Salad

Prep time: 15 minutes | Cook time: 25 minutes | Serves 6

Salad	chiles (from 4½-ounce can)
1 cup uncooked quinoa	1 tablespoon olive oil
1 large onion, chopped (1 cup)	1 can (15 ounces) no-salt-added
1½ cups reduced-sodium chicken broth	black beans, drained, rinsed
1 cup packed fresh cilantro leaves	6 medium plum (Roma) tomatoes, chopped (2 cups)
¼ cup raw unsalted hulled pumpkin seeds (pepitas)	2 tablespoons lime juice
2 cloves garlic, sliced	Garnish
⅛ teaspoon ground cumin	1 avocado, pitted, peeled, thinly sliced
2 tablespoons chopped green	4 small cilantro sprigs

1. Rinse quinoa thoroughly by placing in a fine-mesh strainer and holding under cold running water until water runs clear; drain well. 2. Spray 3-quart saucepan with cooking spray. Heat over medium heat. Add onion to pan; cook 6 to 8 minutes, stirring occasionally, until golden brown. Stir in quinoa and chicken broth. Heat to boiling; reduce heat. Cover and simmer 10 to 15 minutes or until all liquid is absorbed; remove from heat. 3. Meanwhile, in small food processor, place cilantro, pumpkin seeds, garlic and cumin. Cover; process 5 to 10 seconds, using quick on-and-off motions; scrape side. Add chiles and oil. Cover; process, using quick on-and-off motions, until paste forms. 4. To cooked quinoa, add pesto mixture and the remaining salad ingredients. Refrigerate at least 30 minutes to blend flavors. 5. To serve, divide salad evenly among 4 plates; top each serving with 3 or 4 slices avocado and 1 sprig cilantro.

Per Serving:

calorie: 310 | fat: 12g | protein: 13g | carbs: 38g | sugars: 5g | fiber: 9g | sodium: 170mg

Italian Bean Burgers

Prep time: 10 minutes | Cook time: 20 minutes | Makes 9 burgers

2 cans (14 or 15 ounces each) chickpeas, drained and rinsed	Scant ½ teaspoon sea salt
1 medium–large clove garlic, cut in half	2 tablespoons chopped fresh oregano
2 tablespoons tomato paste	⅓ cup roughly chopped fresh basil leaves
1½ tablespoons red wine vinegar (can substitute apple cider vinegar)	1 cup rolled oats
1 tablespoon tahini	⅓ cup chopped sun-dried tomatoes (not packed in oil)
1 teaspoon Dijon mustard	½ cup roughly chopped kalamata or green olives
½ teaspoon onion powder	

1. In a food processor, combine the chickpeas, garlic, tomato paste, vinegar, tahini, mustard, onion powder, and salt. Puree until fully combined. Add the oregano, basil, and oats, and pulse briefly. (You want to combine the ingredients but retain some of the basil's texture.) Finally, pulse in the sun-dried tomatoes and olives, again maintaining some texture. Transfer the mixture to a bowl and refrigerate, covered, for 30 minutes or longer. 2. Preheat the oven to 400°F. Line a baking sheet with parchment paper. Use an ice cream scoop to scoop the mixture onto the prepared baking sheet, flattening to shape into patties. Bake for about 20 minutes, flipping the burgers halfway through. Alternatively, you can cook the burgers in a nonstick skillet over medium heat for 6 to 8 minutes Per side, or until golden brown. Serve.

Per Serving:

calorie: 148 | fat: 4g | protein: 6g | carbs: 23g | sugars: 4g | fiber: 6g | sodium: 387mg

Whole-Wheat Couscous with Pecans

Prep time: 10 minutes | Cook time: 5 minutes | Serves 6

For the Dressing	Pinch sea salt
¼ cup extra-virgin olive oil	1 teaspoon butter
2 tablespoons balsamic vinegar	2 cups boiling water
1 teaspoon honey	1 scallion, white and green parts, chopped
Sea salt	½ cup chopped pecans
Freshly ground black pepper	2 tablespoons chopped fresh parsley
For the Couscous	
1¼ cups whole-wheat couscous	

To Make the Dressing:1. Whisk together the oil, vinegar, and honey. 2. Season with salt and pepper and set it aside.To Make the Couscous: 1. Put the couscous, salt, and butter in a large heat-proof bowl and pour the boiling water on top. Stir and cover the bowl. Let it sit for 5 minutes. Uncover and fluff the couscous with a fork. 2. Stir in the dressing, scallion, pecans, and parsley. 3. Serve warm.

Per Serving:

calorie: 360 | fat: 19g | protein: 8g | carbs: 43g | sugars: 3g | fiber: 6g | sodium: 69mg

Herbed Beans and Brown Rice

Prep time: 15 minutes | Cook time: 15 minutes | Serves 8

2 teaspoons extra-virgin olive oil	red kidney beans, rinsed and drained
½ sweet onion, chopped	1 large tomato, chopped
1 teaspoon minced jalapeño pepper	1 teaspoon chopped fresh thyme
1 teaspoon minced garlic	Sea salt
1 (15 ounces) can sodium-free	Freshly ground black pepper
	2 cups cooked brown rice

1. Place a large skillet over medium-high heat and add the olive oil. 2. Sauté the onion, jalapeño, and garlic until softened, about 3 minutes. 3. Stir in the beans, tomato, and thyme. 4. Cook until heated through, about 10 minutes. Season with salt and pepper. 5. Serve over the warm brown rice.

Per Serving:
calorie: 97 | fat: 2g | protein: 3g | carbs: 18g | sugars: 2g | fiber: 4g | sodium: 20mg

Curried Rice with Pineapple

Prep time: 5 minutes | Cook time: 35 minutes | Serves 8

1 onion, chopped	1 teaspoon curry powder
1½ cups water	1 teaspoon ground turmeric
1¼ cups low-sodium chicken broth	1 teaspoon ground ginger
1 cup uncooked brown basmati rice, soaked in water 20 minutes and drained before cooking	2 garlic cloves, minced
	One 8-ounce can pineapple chunks packed in juice, drained
2 red bell peppers, minced	¼ cup sliced almonds, toasted

1. In a medium saucepan, combine the onion, water, and chicken broth. Bring to a boil, and add the rice, peppers, curry powder, turmeric, ginger, and garlic. Cover, placing a paper towel in between the pot and the lid, and reduce the heat. Simmer for 25 minutes. 2. Add the pineapple, and continue to simmer 5–7 minutes more until rice is tender and water is absorbed. Taste and add salt, if desired. Transfer to a serving bowl, and garnish with almonds to serve.

Per Serving:
calorie: 144 | fat: 3g | protein: 4g | carbs: 27g | sugars: 6g | fiber: 3g | sodium: 16mg

Wild Rice with Blueberries and Pumpkin Seeds

Prep time: 15 minutes | Cook time: 45 minutes | Serves 4

1 tablespoon extra-virgin olive oil	drained
½ sweet onion, chopped	Pinch sea salt
2½ cups sodium-free chicken broth	½ cup toasted pumpkin seeds
	½ cup blueberries
1 cup wild rice, rinsed and	1 teaspoon chopped fresh basil

1. Place a medium saucepan over medium-high heat and add the oil. 2. Sauté the onion until softened and translucent, about 3 minutes.

3. Stir in the broth and bring to a boil. 4. Stir in the rice and salt and reduce the heat to low. Cover and simmer until the rice is tender, about 40 minutes. 5. Drain off any excess broth, if necessary. Stir in the pumpkin seeds, blueberries, and basil. 6. Serve warm.

Per Serving:
calorie: 306 | fat: 15g | protein: 12g | carbs: 37g | sugars: 7g | fiber: 6g | sodium: 12mg

Rice with Spinach and Feta

Prep time: 10 minutes | Cook time: 15 minutes | Serves 4

¾ cup uncooked brown rice	½ teaspoon dried oregano
1½ cups water	9 cups fresh spinach, stems trimmed, washed, patted dry, and coarsely chopped
1 tablespoon extra-virgin olive oil	
1 medium onion, diced	⅓ cup crumbled fat-free feta cheese
1 cup sliced mushrooms	
2 garlic cloves, minced	⅛ teaspoon freshly ground black pepper
1 tablespoon lemon juice	

1. In a medium saucepan over medium heat, combine the rice and water. Bring to a boil, cover, reduce heat, and simmer for 15 minutes. Transfer to a serving bowl. 2. In a skillet, heat the oil. Sauté the onion, mushrooms, and garlic for 5 to 7 minutes. Stir in the lemon juice and oregano. Add the spinach, cheese, and pepper, tossing until the spinach is slightly wilted. 3. Toss with rice and serve.

Per Serving:
calorie: 205 | fat: 5g | protein: 7g | carbs: 34g | sugars: 2g | fiber: 4g | sodium: 129mg

Easy Lentil Burgers

Prep time: 10 minutes | Cook time: 20 minutes | Serves 5

1 medium-large clove garlic	2 teaspoons onion powder
2 tablespoons tamari	¼ teaspoon sea salt
2 tablespoons tomato paste	Few pinches freshly ground black pepper
1 tablespoon red wine vinegar	
1½ tablespoons tahini	3 cups cooked brown lentils
2 tablespoons fresh thyme or oregano	1 cup toasted breadcrumbs
	½ cup rolled oats

1. In a food processor, combine the garlic, tamari, tomato paste, vinegar, tahini, thyme or oregano, onion powder, salt, pepper, and 1½ cups of the lentils. Puree until fairly smooth. Add the breadcrumbs, rolled oats, and the remaining 1½ cups of lentils. Pulse a few times. At this stage you're looking for a sticky texture that will hold together when pressed. If the mixture is still a little crumbly, pulse a few more times. 2. Preheat the oven to 400°F. Line a baking sheet with parchment paper. 3. Use an ice cream scoop to scoop the mixture onto the prepared baking sheet, flattening to shape into patties. Bake for about 20 minutes, flipping the burgers halfway through. Alternatively, you can cook the burgers in a nonstick skillet over medium heat for 4 to 5 minutes Per side, or until golden brown.

Per Serving:
calorie: 148 | fat: 2g | protein: 8g | carbs: 24g | sugars: 1g | fiber: 5g | sodium: 369mg

Prep time: 20 minutes | Cook time: 10 minutes | Serves 4

Salad

½ cup uncooked whole wheat couscous

1½ cups water

¼ teaspoon salt

1 can (15 oz) chickpeas (garbanzo beans), drained, rinsed

1 can (14½ oz) diced tomatoes with green chiles, undrained

½ cup frozen shelled edamame (green soybeans) or lima beans, thawed

2 tablespoons chopped fresh cilantro

Green bell peppers, halved, if desired

Dressing

2 tablespoons olive oil

1 teaspoon ground coriander

½ teaspoon ground cumin

½ teaspoon ground cinnamon

1. Cook couscous in the water and salt as directed on package. 2. Meanwhile, in medium bowl, mix chickpeas, tomatoes, edamame and cilantro. In small bowl, mix dressing ingredients until well blended. 3. Add cooked couscous to salad; mix well. Pour dressing over salad; stir gently to mix. Spoon salad mixture into halved bell peppers. Serve immediately, or cover and refrigerate until serving time.

Per Serving:

calorie: 370 | fat: 11g | protein: 16g | carbs: 53g | sugars: 6g | fiber: 10g | sodium: 460mg

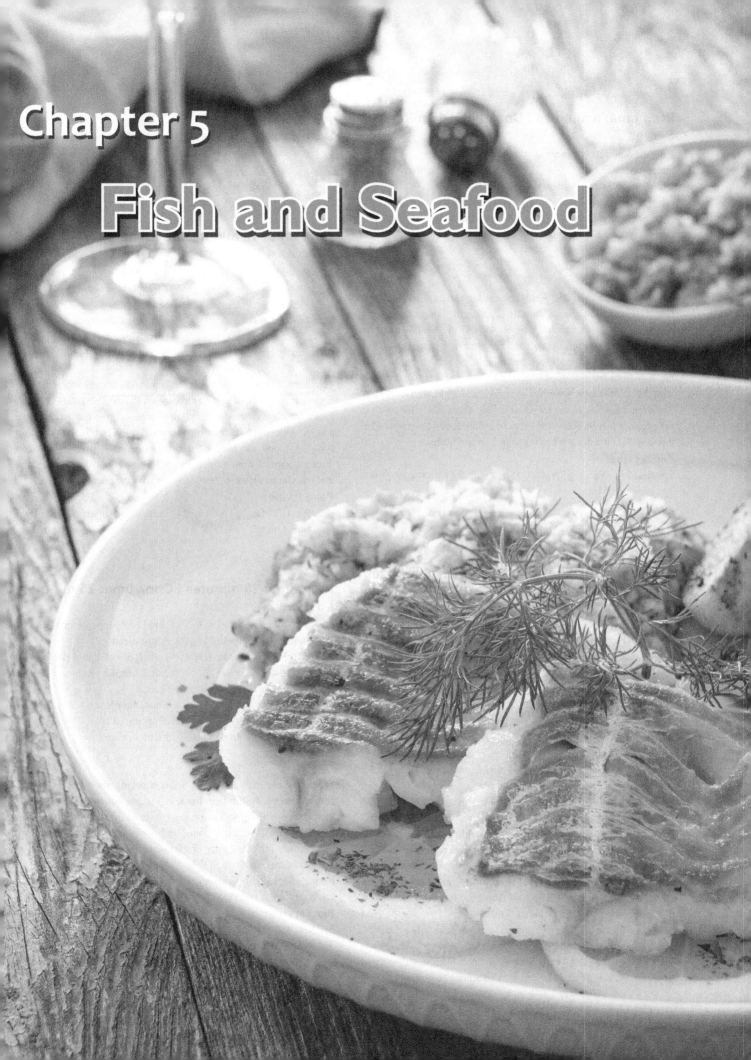

Chapter 5
Fish and Seafood

Sesame-Crusted Halibut

Prep time: 5 minutes | Cook time: 15 minutes | Serves 2

1 tablespoon freshly squeezed lemon juice	halved
1 tablespoon extra-virgin olive oil	2 tablespoons sesame seeds, toasted
1 garlic clove, minced	1 teaspoon dried basil
Freshly ground black pepper, to season	1 teaspoon dried marjoram
	½ cup minced chives
1 (8 ounces) halibut fillet,	⅛ teaspoon salt
	2 lemon wedges

1. Preheat the oven to 450°F. 2. Line a baking sheet with aluminum foil. 3. In a shallow glass dish, mix together the lemon juice, olive oil, and garlic. Season with pepper. 4. Add the halibut and turn to coat. Cover and refrigerate for 15 minutes. 5. In a small bowl, combine the sesame seeds, basil, marjoram, and chives. 6. Remove the fish from the refrigerator. Sprinkle with the salt. Coat evenly with the sesame seed mixture, covering the sides as well as the top. 7. Transfer the fish to the prepared baking sheet. Place the sheet in the preheated oven. Roast for 10 to 14 minutes, or until just cooked through. 8. Garnish each serving with 1 lemon wedge.

Per Serving:

calories: 331 | fat: 27g | protein: 18g | carbs: 3g | sugars: 0g | fiber: 2g | sodium: 251mg

Walnut-Crusted Halibut with Pear Salad

Prep time: 10 minutes | Cook time: 10 minutes | Serves 4

For the halibut	oil
¾ cup finely chopped toasted walnuts	For the salad
2 tablespoons bread crumbs	6 cups packed mixed greens
¼ cup chopped fresh parsley	1 pear, thinly sliced
2 tablespoons chopped fresh chives	¼ cup chopped fresh parsley
	¼ cup chopped fresh chives
4 (6 to 8 ounces) halibut fillets	Zest and juice of 1 lemon
Kosher salt	Extra-virgin olive oil, for the dressing
Freshly ground black pepper	Kosher salt
1 tablespoon extra-virgin olive	Freshly ground black pepper

To make the halibut 1. Preheat the broiler. Line a baking sheet with parchment paper. 2. In a small bowl, combine the walnuts, bread crumbs, parsley, and chives. 3. Pat the halibut fillets dry, season them with salt and pepper and rub ½ tablespoon of extra-virgin olive oil on each fillet. Place the fillets on the prepared baking sheet. Sprinkle the walnut mixture evenly on top of each fillet and press slightly, so the topping will stick. 4. Broil the fish until the crust is golden and the fish is fully cooked, 5 to 8 minutes. To make the salad 5. Meanwhile, in a large bowl, toss the greens, pear, parsley, chives, and zest until well combined. Drizzle the salad with the lemon juice and a bit of extra-virgin olive oil to taste. Season with salt and pepper to taste. 6. Evenly divide the salad among four plates and top

with the fish. Serve. 7. Store any leftovers in an airtight container in the refrigerator for up to 2 days.

Per Serving:

calories: 551 | fat: 43g | protein: 31g | carbs: 13g | sugars: 4g | fiber: 5g | sodium: 196mg

Haddock with Creamy Cucumber Sauce

Prep time: 10 minutes | Cook time: 10 minutes | Serves 4

¼ cup 2 percent plain Greek yogurt	2 teaspoons chopped fresh mint
	1 teaspoon honey
½ English cucumber, grated, liquid squeezed out	Sea salt
	4 (5-ounce) haddock fillets
½ scallion, white and green parts, finely chopped	Freshly ground black pepper
	Nonstick cooking spray

1. In a small bowl, stir together the yogurt, cucumber, scallion, mint, honey, and a pinch of salt. Set it aside. 2. Pat the fish fillets dry with paper towels and season them lightly with salt and pepper. 3. Place a large skillet over medium-high heat and spray lightly with cooking spray. 4. Cook the haddock, turning once, until it is just cooked through, about 5 minutes per side. 5. Remove the fish from the heat and transfer to plates. 6. Serve topped with the cucumber sauce.

Per Serving:

calories: 123 | fat: 1g | protein: 24g | carbs: 3g | sugars: 3g | fiber: 0g | sodium: 310mg

Whole Veggie-Stuffed Trout

Prep time: 10 minutes | Cook time: 25 minutes | Serves 2

Nonstick cooking spray	½ red bell pepper, seeded and thinly sliced
2 (8-ounce) whole trout fillets, dressed (cleaned but with bones and skin intact)	1 small onion, thinly sliced
	2 or 3 shiitake mushrooms, sliced
1 tablespoon extra-virgin olive oil	1 poblano pepper, seeded and thinly sliced
¼ teaspoon salt	
⅛ teaspoon freshly ground black pepper	1 lemon, sliced

1. Preheat the oven to 425°F. Spray a baking sheet with nonstick cooking spray. 2. Rub both trout, inside and out, with the olive oil, then season with the salt and pepper. 3. In a large bowl, combine the bell pepper, onion, mushrooms, and poblano pepper. Stuff half of this mixture into the cavity of each fish. Top the mixture with 2 or 3 lemon slices inside each fish. 4. Arrange the fish on the prepared baking sheet side by side and roast for 25 minutes until the fish is cooked through and the vegetables are tender.

Per Serving:

calories: 452 | fat: 22g | protein: 49g | carbs: 14g | sugars: 2g | fiber: 3g | sodium: 357mg

Bacon-Wrapped Scallops

Prep time: 5 minutes | Cook time: 10 minutes | Serves 4

8 (1-ounce / 28-g) sea scallops, cleaned and patted dry	¼ teaspoon salt
	¼ teaspoon ground black pepper
8 slices sugar-free bacon	

1. Wrap each scallop in 1 slice bacon and secure with a toothpick. Sprinkle with salt and pepper. 2. Place scallops into ungreased air fryer basket. Adjust the temperature to 360ºF (182ºC) and air fry for 10 minutes. Scallops will be opaque and firm, and have an internal temperature of 135ºF (57ºC) when done. Serve warm.

Per Serving:
calories: 251 | fat: 21g | protein: 13g | carbs: 2g | sugars: 0g | fiber: 0g | sodium: 612mg

Salmon Florentine

Prep time: 10 minutes | Cook time: 30 minutes | Serves 4

1 teaspoon extra-virgin olive oil	removed, torn into 3-inch pieces
½ sweet onion, finely chopped	Sea salt
1 teaspoon minced garlic	Freshly ground black pepper
3 cups baby spinach	4 (5-ounce) salmon fillets
1 cup kale, tough stems	Lemon wedges, for serving

1. Preheat the oven to 350°F. 2. Place a large skillet over medium-high heat and add the oil. 3. Sauté the onion and garlic until softened and translucent, about 3 minutes. 4. Add the spinach and kale and sauté until the greens wilt, about 5 minutes. 5. Remove the skillet from the heat and season the greens with salt and pepper. 6. Place the salmon fillets so they are nestled in the greens and partially covered by them. Bake the salmon until it is opaque, about 20 minutes. 7. Serve immediately with a squeeze of fresh lemon.

Per Serving:
calories: 211 | fat: 8g | protein: 30g | carbs: 5g | sugars: 2g | fiber: 1g | sodium: 129mg

Poached Red Snapper

Prep time: 5 minutes | Cook time: 25 minutes | Serves 4

1 cup dry white wine	¼ teaspoon salt
1 medium lemon, sliced	1 cup water
6 parsley sprigs, plus additional for garnish	1 red snapper (about 1½ to 2 pounds), cleaned and scaled
5 peppercorns	with head and tail left on
5 scallions, sliced	1 lemon, sliced
2 bay leaves	

1. In a fish poacher or very large skillet, combine the wine, lemon slices, 6 parsley sprigs, peppercorns, scallions, bay leaves, salt, and water. Bring the mixture to a boil; add the snapper. 2. Cover the pan, lower the heat, and simmer the red snapper for 15–20 minutes until the fish flakes easily with a fork. 3. Carefully lift out the snapper, and transfer to a platter. Garnish with lemon slices and parsley.

Per Serving:
calories: 269 | fat: 3g | protein: 43g | carbs: 6g | sugars: 2g | fiber: 2g | sodium: 285mg

Tilapia with Pecans

Prep time: 20 minutes | Cook time: 16 minutes | Serves 5

2 tablespoons ground flaxseeds	2 tablespoons extra-virgin olive oil
1 teaspoon paprika	
Sea salt and white pepper, to taste	½ cup pecans, ground
	5 tilapia fillets, sliced into halves
1 teaspoon garlic paste	

1. Combine the ground flaxseeds, paprika, salt, white pepper, garlic paste, olive oil, and ground pecans in a Ziploc bag. Add the fish fillets and shake to coat well. 2. Spritz the air fryer basket with cooking spray. Cook in the preheated air fryer at 400ºF (204ºC) for 10 minutes; turn them over and cook for 6 minutes more. Work in batches. 3. Serve with lemon wedges, if desired. Enjoy!

Per Serving:
calorie: 344 | fat: 23g | protein: 28g | carbs: 6g | sugars: 1g | fiber: 4g | sodium: 81mg

Spicy Shrimp Fajitas

Prep time: 30 minutes | Cook time: 20 minutes | Makes 6 fajitas

Marinade	medium shrimp, thawed if frozen, tail shells removed
1 tablespoon lime juice	
1 tablespoon olive or canola oil	2 medium red bell peppers, cut into strips (2 cups)
¼ teaspoon salt	
1 teaspoon chili powder	1 medium red onion, sliced (2 cups)
1 teaspoon ground cumin	
2 cloves garlic, crushed	Olive oil cooking spray
Pinch ground red pepper (cayenne)	6 flour tortillas (8 inch)
	¾ cup refrigerated guacamole (from 14-oz package)
Fajitas	
2 lb uncooked deveined peeled	

1. Heat gas or charcoal grill. In 1-gallon resealable food-storage plastic bag, mix marinade ingredients. Add shrimp; seal bag and toss to coat. Set aside while grilling vegetables, turning bag once. 2. In medium bowl, place bell peppers and onion; spray with cooking spray. Place vegetables in grill basket (grill "wok"). Wrap tortillas in foil; set aside. 3. Place basket on grill rack over medium heat. Cover grill; cook 10 minutes, turning vegetables once. 4. Drain shrimp; discard marinade. Add shrimp to grill basket. Cover grill; cook 5 to 7 minutes longer, turning shrimp and vegetables once, until shrimp are pink. Place wrapped tortillas on grill. Cook 2 minutes, turning once, until warm. 5. On each tortilla, place shrimp, vegetables and guacamole; fold tortilla over filling.

Per Serving:
calories: 310 | fat: 10g | protein: 27g | carbs: 29g | sugars: 4g | fiber: 2g | sodium: 770mg

Marinated Swordfish Skewers

Prep time: 30 minutes | Cook time: 6 to 8 minutes | Serves 4

1 pound (454 g) filleted swordfish	parsley
¼ cup avocado oil	2 teaspoons Dijon mustard
2 tablespoons freshly squeezed lemon juice	Sea salt and freshly ground black pepper, to taste
1 tablespoon minced fresh	3 ounces (85 g) cherry tomatoes

1. Cut the fish into 1½-inch chunks, picking out any remaining bones. 2. In a large bowl, whisk together the oil, lemon juice, parsley, and Dijon mustard. Season to taste with salt and pepper. Add the fish and toss to coat the pieces. Cover and marinate the fish chunks in the refrigerator for 30 minutes. 3. Remove the fish from the marinade. Thread the fish and cherry tomatoes on 4 skewers, alternating as you go. 4. Set the air fryer to 400ºF (204ºC). Place the skewers in the air fryer basket and air fry for 3 minutes. Flip the skewers and cook for 3 to 5 minutes longer, until the fish is cooked through and an instant-read thermometer reads 140ºF (60ºC).

Per Serving:

calories: 291 | fat: 21g | protein: 23g | carbs: 2g | sugars: 1g | fiber: 0g | sodium: 121mg

Salade Niçoise with Oil-Packed Tuna

Prep time: 5 minutes | Cook time: 20 minutes | Serves 4

8 ounces small red potatoes, quartered	¼ teaspoon fine sea salt
8 ounces green beans, trimmed	1 tablespoon minced shallot
4 large eggs	2 hearts romaine lettuce, leaves separated and torn into bite-size pieces
french vinaigrette	
2 tablespoons extra-virgin olive oil	½ cup grape tomatoes, halved
2 tablespoons cold-pressed avocado oil	¼ cup pitted Niçoise or Greek olives
2 tablespoons white wine vinegar	One 7 ounces can oil-packed tuna, drained and flaked
1 tablespoon water	Freshly ground black pepper
1 teaspoon Dijon mustard	1 tablespoon chopped fresh flat-leaf parsley
½ teaspoon dried oregano	

1. Pour 1 cup water into the Instant Pot and place a steamer basket into the pot. Add the potatoes, green beans, and eggs to the basket. 2. Secure the lid and set the Pressure Release to Sealing. Select the Steam setting and set the cooking time for 3 minutes at high pressure. (The pot will take about 15 minutes to come up to pressure before the cooking program begins.) 3. To make the vinaigrette: While the vegetables and eggs are steaming, in a small jar or other small container with a tight-fitting lid, combine the olive oil, avocado oil, vinegar, water, mustard, oregano, salt, and shallot and shake vigorously to emulsify. Set aside. 4. Prepare an ice bath. 5. When the cooking program ends, perform a quick release by moving the Pressure Release to Venting. Open the pot and, wearing heat-resistant mitts, lift out the steamer basket. Using tongs, transfer the eggs and green beans to the ice bath, leaving the potatoes in the steamer basket. 6. While the eggs and green beans are cooling, divide the lettuce, tomatoes, olives, and tuna among four shallow individual bowls. Drain the eggs and green beans. Peel and halve the eggs lengthwise, then arrange them on the salads along with the green beans and potatoes. 7. Spoon the vinaigrette over the salads and sprinkle with the pepper and parsley. Serve right away.

Per Serving:

calories: 367 | fat: 23g | protein: 20g | carbs: 23g | sugars: 7g | fiber: 4g | sodium: 268mg

Herb-Crusted Halibut

Prep time: 10 minutes | Cook time: 20 minutes | Serves 4

4 (5-ounce) halibut fillets	parsley
Extra-virgin olive oil, for brushing	1 teaspoon chopped fresh thyme
½ cup coarsely ground unsalted pistachios	1 teaspoon chopped fresh basil
	Pinch sea salt
1 tablespoon chopped fresh	Pinch freshly ground black pepper

1. Preheat the oven to 350°F. 2. Line a baking sheet with parchment paper. 3. Pat the halibut fillets dry with a paper towel and place them on the baking sheet. 4. Brush the halibut generously with olive oil. 5. In a small bowl, stir together the pistachios, parsley, thyme, basil, salt, and pepper. 6. Spoon the nut and herb mixture evenly on the fish, spreading it out so the tops of the fillets are covered. 7. Bake the halibut until it flakes when pressed with a fork, about 20 minutes. 8. Serve immediately.

Per Serving:

calories: 351 | fat: 27g | protein: 24g | carbs: 4g | sugars: 1g | fiber: 2g | sodium: 214mg

Crab-Stuffed Avocado Boats

Prep time: 5 minutes | Cook time: 7 minutes | Serves 4

2 medium avocados, halved and pitted	¼ teaspoon Old Bay seasoning
8 ounces (227 g) cooked crab meat	2 tablespoons peeled and diced yellow onion
	2 tablespoons mayonnaise

1. Scoop out avocado flesh in each avocado half, leaving ½ inch around edges to form a shell. Chop scooped-out avocado. 2. In a medium bowl, combine crab meat, Old Bay seasoning, onion, mayonnaise, and chopped avocado. Place ¼ mixture into each avocado shell. 3. Place avocado boats into ungreased air fryer basket. Adjust the temperature to 350ºF (177ºC) and air fry for 7 minutes. Avocado will be browned on the top and mixture will be bubbling when done. Serve warm.

Per Serving:

calories: 226 | fat: 17g | protein: 12g | carbs: 10g | sugars: 1g | fiber: 7g | sodium: 239mg

Almond Pesto Salmon

Prep time: 5 minutes | Cook time: 12 minutes | Serves 2

¼ cup pesto	(about 4 ounces / 113 g each)
¼ cup sliced almonds, roughly chopped	2 tablespoons unsalted butter, melted
2 (1½-inch-thick) salmon fillets	

1. In a small bowl, mix pesto and almonds. Set aside. 2. Place fillets into a round baking dish. 3. Brush each fillet with butter and place half of the pesto mixture on the top of each fillet. Place dish into the air fryer basket. 4. Adjust the temperature to 390°F (199°C) and set the timer for 12 minutes. 5. Salmon will easily flake when fully cooked and reach an internal temperature of at least 145°F (63°C). Serve warm.

Per Serving:

calories: 478 | fat: 39g | protein: 29g | carbs: 4g | sugars: 1g | fiber: 2g | sodium: 366mg

Baked Garlic Scampi

Prep time: 5 minutes | Cook time: 10 minutes | Serves 4

1 tablespoon extra-virgin olive oil	parsley, divided
¼ teaspoon salt	1 pound large shrimp, shelled (with tails left on) and deveined
7 garlic cloves, crushed	Juice and zest of 1 lemon
2 tablespoons chopped fresh	2 cups baby arugula

1. Preheat the oven to 350 degrees. Grease a 13-x-9-x-2-inch baking pan with the olive oil. Add the salt, garlic, and 1 tablespoon of the parsley in a medium bowl; mix well, and set aside. 2. Arrange the shrimp in a single layer in the baking pan, and bake for 3 minutes, uncovered. Turn the shrimp, and sprinkle with the lemon peel, lemon juice, and the remaining 1 tablespoon of parsley. Continue to bake 1–2 minutes more until the shrimp are bright pink and tender. 3. Remove the shrimp from the oven. Place the arugula on a serving platter, and top with the shrimp. Spoon the garlic mixture over the shrimp and arugula, and serve.

Per Serving:

calories: 140 | fat: 4g | protein: 23g | carbs: 3g | sugars: 1g | fiber: 0g | sodium: 285mg

Cobia with Lemon-Caper Sauce

Prep time: 25 minutes | Cook time: 10 minutes | Serves 4

⅓ cup all-purpose flour	½ cup reduced-sodium chicken broth
¼ teaspoon salt	
¼ teaspoon pepper	2 tablespoons lemon juice
1¼ lb cobia or sea bass fillets, cut into 4 pieces	1 tablespoon capers, rinsed, drained
2 tablespoons olive oil	1 tablespoon chopped fresh parsley
⅓ cup dry white wine	

1. In shallow dish, stir flour, salt and pepper. Coat cobia pieces in flour mixture (reserve remaining flour mixture). In 12-inch nonstick skillet, heat oil over medium-high heat. Place coated cobia in oil. Cook 8 to 10 minutes, turning halfway through cooking, until fish flakes easily with fork; remove from heat. Lift fish from skillet to serving platter with slotted spatula (do not discard drippings); keep warm. 2. Heat skillet (with drippings) over medium heat. Stir in 1 tablespoon reserved flour mixture; cook and stir 30 seconds. Stir in wine; cook about 30 seconds or until thickened and slightly reduced. Stir in chicken broth and lemon juice; cook and stir 1 to 2 minutes until sauce is smooth and slightly thickened. Stir in capers. 3. Serve sauce over cobia; sprinkle with parsley.

Per Serving:

calories: 230 | fat: 9g | protein: 28g | carbs: 9g | sugars: 0g | fiber: 0g | sodium: 400mg

Easy Tuna Patties

Prep time: 5 minutes | Cook time: 10 minutes | Serves 4

1 pound canned tuna, drained	1 tablespoon chopped fresh dill
1 cup whole-wheat bread crumbs	Juice and zest of 1 lemon
2 large eggs, beaten	3 tablespoons extra-virgin olive oil
½ onion, grated	½ cup tartar sauce, for serving

1. In a large bowl, combine the tuna, bread crumbs, eggs, onion, dill, and lemon juice and zest. Form the mixture into 4 patties and chill for 10 minutes. 2. In a large nonstick skillet over medium-high heat, heat the olive oil until it shimmers. Add the patties and cook until browned on both sides, 4 to 5 minutes per side. 3. Serve topped with the tartar sauce.

Per Serving:

calories: 473 | fat: 25g | protein: 34g | carbs: 27g | sugars: 4g | fiber: 2g | sodium: 479mg

Tomato Tuna Melts

Prep time: 5 minutes | Cook time: 5 minutes | Serves 2

1 (5-ounce) can chunk light tuna packed in water, drained	celery
	1 tablespoon finely chopped red onion
2 tablespoons plain nonfat Greek yogurt	Pinch cayenne pepper
2 teaspoons freshly squeezed lemon juice	1 large tomato, cut into ¾-inch-thick rounds
2 tablespoons finely chopped	½ cup shredded cheddar cheese

1. Preheat the broiler to high. 2. In a medium bowl, combine the tuna, yogurt, lemon juice, celery, red onion, and cayenne pepper. Stir well. 3. Arrange the tomato slices on a baking sheet. Top each with some tuna salad and cheddar cheese. 4. Broil for 3 to 4 minutes until the cheese is melted and bubbly. Serve.

Per Serving:

calories: 243 | fat: 10g | protein: 30g | carbs: 7g | sugars: 2g | fiber: 1g | sodium: 444mg

Air Fryer Fish Fry

Prep time: 5 minutes | Cook time: 15 minutes | Serves 4

2 cups low-fat buttermilk	½ cup plain yellow cornmeal
½ teaspoon garlic powder	½ cup chickpea flour
½ teaspoon onion powder	¼ teaspoon cayenne pepper
4 (4 ounces) flounder fillets	Freshly ground black pepper

1. In a large bowl, combine the buttermilk, garlic powder, and onion powder. 2. Add the flounder, turning until well coated, and set aside to marinate for 20 minutes. 3. In a shallow bowl, stir the cornmeal, chickpea flour, cayenne, and pepper together. 4. Dredge the fillets in the meal mixture, turning until well coated. Place in the basket of an air fryer. 5. Set the air fryer to 380°F, close, and cook for 12 minutes.

Per Serving:

calories: 266 | fat: 7g | protein: 27g | carbs: 24g | sugars: 8g | fiber: 2g | sodium: 569mg

Asian Cod with Brown Rice, Asparagus, and Mushrooms

Prep time: 5 minutes | Cook time: 25 minutes | Serves 2

¾ cup Minute brand brown rice	2 green onions, white and green parts, thinly sliced
½ cup water	
Two 5-ounce skinless cod fillets	12 ounces asparagus, trimmed
1 tablespoon soy sauce or tamari	4 ounces shiitake mushrooms, stems removed and sliced
1 tablespoon fresh lemon juice	
½ teaspoon peeled and grated fresh ginger	⅛ teaspoon fine sea salt
	⅛ teaspoon freshly ground black pepper
1 tablespoon extra-virgin olive oil or 1 tablespoon unsalted butter, cut into 8 pieces	Lemon wedges for serving

1. Pour 1 cup water into the Instant Pot. Have ready two-tier stackable stainless-steel containers. 2. In one of the containers, combine the rice and ½ cup water, then gently shake the container to spread the rice into an even layer, making sure all of the grains are submerged. Place the fish fillets on top of the rice. In a small bowl, stir together the soy sauce, lemon juice, and ginger. Pour the soy sauce mixture over the fillets. Drizzle 1 teaspoon olive oil on each fillet (or top with two pieces of the butter), and sprinkle the green onions on and around the fish. 3. In the second container, arrange the asparagus in the center in as even a layer as possible. Place the mushrooms on either side of the asparagus. Drizzle with the remaining 2 teaspoons olive oil (or put the remaining six pieces butter on top of the asparagus, spacing them evenly). Sprinkle the salt and pepper evenly over the vegetables. 4. Place the container with the rice and fish on the bottom and the vegetable container on top. Cover the top container with its lid and then latch the containers together. Grasping the handle, lower the containers into the Instant Pot. 5. Secure the lid and set the Pressure Release to Sealing. Select the Pressure Cook or Manual setting and set the cooking time for 15 minutes at high pressure. (The pot will take about 10 minutes to come up to pressure before the cooking program begins.) 6. When the cooking program ends, let the pressure release naturally for 5 minutes, then move the Pressure Release to Venting to release any remaining steam. Open the pot and, wearing heat-resistant mitts, lift out the stacked containers. Unlatch, unstack, and open the containers, taking care not to get burned by the steam. 7. Transfer the vegetables, rice, and fish to plates and serve right away, with the lemon wedges on the side.

Per Serving:

calories: 344 | fat: 11g | protein: 27g | carbs: 46g | sugars: 6g | fiber: 7g | sodium: 637mg

Calypso Shrimp with Black Bean Salsa

Prep time: 25 minutes | Cook time: 5 minutes | Serves 4

Shrimp	1 medium mango, peeled, pitted and chopped (1 cup)
½ teaspoon grated lime peel	
1 tablespoon lime juice	1 small red bell pepper, chopped (½ cup)
1 tablespoon canola oil	
1 teaspoon finely chopped gingerroot	2 medium green onions, sliced (2 tablespoons)
1 clove garlic, finely chopped	1 tablespoon chopped fresh cilantro
1 pound uncooked deveined peeled large shrimp, thawed if frozen	
	½ teaspoon grated lime peel
Salsa	1 to 2 tablespoons lime juice
1 can (15 ounces) black beans, drained, rinsed	1 tablespoon red wine vinegar
	¼ teaspoon ground red pepper (cayenne)

1. In medium glass or plastic bowl, mix lime peel, lime juice, oil, gingerroot and garlic. Stir in shrimp; let stand 15 minutes. 2. Meanwhile, in medium bowl, mix salsa ingredients. 3. In 10-inch skillet, cook shrimp over medium-high heat about 5 minutes, turning once, until pink. Serve with salsa.

Per Serving:

calories: 300| fat: 5g | protein: 26g | carbs: 37g | sugars: 7g | fiber: 12g | sodium: 190mg

Grilled Rosemary Swordfish

Prep time: 5 minutes | Cook time: 15 minutes | Serves 4

2 scallions, thinly sliced	1 teaspoon fresh rosemary, finely chopped
2 tablespoons extra-virgin olive oil	
	4 swordfish steaks (1 pound total)
2 tablespoons white wine vinegar	

1. In a small bowl, combine the scallions, olive oil, vinegar, and rosemary. Pour over the swordfish steaks. Let the steaks marinate for 30 minutes. 2. Remove the steaks from the marinade, and grill for 5–7 minutes per side, brushing with marinade. Transfer to a serving platter, and serve.

Per Serving:

calories: 225 | fat: 14g | protein: 22g | carbs: 0g | sugars: 0g | fiber: 0g | sodium: 92mg

Roasted Tilapia and Vegetables

Prep time: 15 minutes | Cook time: 20 minutes | Serves 4

½ pound fresh asparagus spears, trimmed, halved
2 small zucchini, halved lengthwise, cut into ½-inch pieces
1 red bell pepper, cut into ½-inch strips
1 large onion, cut into ½-inch wedges
1 tablespoon olive oil
2 teaspoons Montreal steak seasoning
4 tilapia fillets (about 1½ pounds)
2 teaspoons butter or margarine, melted
½ teaspoon paprika

1. Heat oven to 450°F. In large bowl, toss asparagus, zucchini, bell pepper, onion and oil. Sprinkle with 1 teaspoon of the steak seasoning; toss to coat. Spread vegetables in ungreased 15x10x1-inch pan. Place on lower oven rack; roast 5 minutes. 2. Meanwhile, spray 13x9-inch (3-quart) glass baking dish with cooking spray. Pat tilapia fillets dry with paper towels. Brush with butter; sprinkle with remaining 1 teaspoon steak seasoning and the paprika. Place in baking dish. 3. Place baking dish on middle oven rack. Roast fish and vegetables 17 to 18 minutes longer or until fish flakes easily with fork and vegetables are tender.

Per Serving:

calories: 250 | fat: 8g | protein: 35g | carbs: 10g | sugars: 5g | fiber: 3g | sodium: 160mg

Lemon-Pepper Salmon with Roasted Broccoli

Prep time: 5 minutes | Cook time: 20 minutes | Serves 4

4 (6 ounces [170 g]) salmon fillets
Cooking oil spray, as needed
Juice of 1 medium lemon (see Tips)
½ teaspoon black pepper
¼ teaspoon garlic salt or ¼ teaspoon sea salt mixed with ¼ teaspoon garlic powder
1 pound (454 g) broccoli florets
¼ teaspoon sea salt
¼ teaspoon garlic powder

1. Preheat the oven to 400°F (204°C). Line two large baking sheets with parchment paper. 2. Place the salmon on the first prepared baking sheet, making sure the fillets are evenly spaced. Spray the salmon with the cooking oil spray. Drizzle the lemon juice over each of the salmon fillets, then sprinkle the black pepper and garlic salt over each fillet. 3. Spread the broccoli out evenly on the second prepared baking sheet and spray the broccoli with cooking oil spray. Sprinkle the sea salt and garlic powder over the broccoli. 4. Place both baking sheets in the oven. Bake the salmon for 10 to 12 minutes, until it is light brown, depending on your preferred doneness and the thickness of the fillets. Bake the broccoli for 12 minutes, until the edges are slightly crispy. Serve the salmon and broccoli immediately.

Per Serving:

calorie: 353 | fat: 19g | protein: 37g | carbs: 9g | sugars: 2g | fiber: 3g | sodium: 406mg

Blackened Pollock

Prep time: 15 minutes | Cook time: 10 minutes | Serves 2

8 ounces pollock (or other white fish) fillet, skinned and halved
3 teaspoons extra-virgin olive oil, divided
1 teaspoon blackening seasoning, or Cajun seasoning, divided
¼ cup thinly sliced onion
4 cups baby spinach, divided
½ small grapefruit, peeled and segmented
2 tablespoons shaved fennel
2 tablespoons pepitas
½ small avocado, peeled, pitted, and sliced, divided

1. Brush both sides of each pollock half with 1½ teaspoons of olive oil. 2. Rub each half all over with ½ teaspoon of blackening seasoning. 3. In a large heavy skillet set over high heat, cook the pollock and onions for 2 to 3 minutes, until blackened. Turn the fillets. Cook for 2 to 3 minutes more, or until blackened and the fish flakes easily with a fork. 4. Put 2 cups of arugula on each serving plate. Top each with 1 pollock half. 5. Top each serving with half of the grapefruit, fennel, pepitas, and avocado.

Per Serving:

calories: 302 | fat: 19g | protein: 20g | carbs: 16g | sugars: 5g | fiber: 8g | sodium: 436mg

North Carolina Fish Stew

Prep time: 20 minutes | Cook time: 20 minutes | Serves 8

½ cup store-bought low-sodium seafood broth
2 large white onions, chopped
4 garlic cloves, minced
¼ cup tomato paste
1 teaspoon red pepper flakes
2 teaspoons smoked paprika
3 bay leaves
1 pound new potatoes, halved
3 cups water
2 pounds fish fillets, such as rockfish, striped bass, or cod, cut into ½- to 1-inch dice
8 medium eggs

1. Select the Sauté setting on an electric pressure cooker, and combine the broth, onions, garlic, tomato paste, red pepper flakes, paprika, and bay leaves. Cook for 2 minutes, or until the onions and garlic are translucent. 2. Add the potatoes and 1 cup of water. 3. Close and lock the lid, and set the pressure valve to sealing. 4. Change to the Manual/Pressure Cook setting, and cook for 3 minutes. 5. Once cooking is complete, quick-release the pressure. Carefully remove the lid. 6. Add the fish and enough of the water just to cover the fish. 7. Close and lock the lid, and set the pressure valve to sealing. 8. Select the Manual/Pressure Cook setting, and cook for 3 more minutes. 9. Once cooking is complete, quick-release the pressure. Carefully remove the lid. 10. Carefully crack the eggs one by one into the stew, keeping the yolks intact. 11. Close and lock the lid, and set the pressure valve to sealing. 12. Select the Manual/Pressure Cook setting, and cook for 1 minute. 13. Once cooking is complete, quick-release the pressure. Carefully remove the lid, discard the bay leaves, and serve in bowls.

Per Serving:

calories: 228 | fat: 5g | protein: 28g | carbs: 16g | sugars: 3g | fiber: 3g | sodium: 184mg

Quinoa Pilaf with Salmon and Asparagus

Prep time: 30 minutes | Cook time: 15 minutes | Serves 4

1 cup uncooked quinoa	1 cup frozen sweet peas (from 1 pound bag), thawed
6 cups water	
1 vegetable bouillon cube	½ cup halved grape tomatoes
1 pound salmon fillets	½ cup vegetable or chicken broth
2 teaspoons butter or margarine	
20 stalks fresh asparagus, cut diagonally into 2-inch pieces (2 cups)	1 teaspoon lemon-pepper seasoning
	2 teaspoons chopped fresh or ½ teaspoon dried dill weed
4 medium green onions, sliced (¼ cup)	

1. Rinse quinoa thoroughly by placing in a fine-mesh strainer and holding under cold running water until water runs clear; drain well. 2. In 2-quart saucepan, heat 2 cups of the water to boiling over high heat. Add quinoa; reduce heat to low. Cover; simmer 10 to 12 minutes or until water is absorbed. 3. Meanwhile, in 12-inch skillet, heat remaining 4 cups water and the bouillon cube to boiling over high heat. Add salmon, skin side up; reduce heat to low. Cover; simmer 10 to 12 minutes or until fish flakes easily with fork. Transfer with slotted spoon to plate; let cool. Discard water. Remove skin from salmon; break into large pieces. 4. Meanwhile, rinse and dry skillet. Melt butter in skillet over medium heat. Add asparagus; cook 5 minutes, stirring frequently. Stir in onions; cook 1 minute, stirring frequently. Stir in peas, tomatoes and broth; cook 1 minute. 5. Gently stir quinoa, salmon, lemon-pepper seasoning and dill weed into asparagus mixture. Cover; cook about 2 minutes or until hot.

Per Serving:
calories: 380 | fat: 12g | protein: 32g | carbs: 37g | sugars: 7g | fiber: 6g | sodium: 600mg

Lobster Fricassee

Prep time: 5 minutes | Cook time: 20 minutes | Serves 4

2 cups shelled lobster meat	¼ teaspoon paprika
1 tablespoon extra-virgin olive oil	¼ teaspoon salt
	⅛ teaspoon freshly ground black pepper
¾ pound mushrooms, sliced	
1 small onion, minced	2 cups cooked whole-wheat pasta
½ cup fat-free milk	
¼ cup flour	¼ cup finely chopped parsley

1. Cut the lobster meat into bite-size pieces. In a saucepan, heat the oil; add the mushrooms and onion, and sauté for 5 to 6 minutes. 2. In a small bowl, whisk the milk and flour, whisking quickly to eliminate any lumps. Pour the milk mixture into the mushroom mixture; mix thoroughly, and continue cooking for 3 to 5 minutes. 3. Add the lobster, paprika, salt, and pepper; continue cooking for 5 to 10 minutes until the lobster is heated through. 4. Spread the pasta onto a serving platter, spoon the lobster and sauce over the top, and garnish with parsley to serve.

Per Serving:
calories: 248 | fat: 5g | protein: 22g | carbs: 31g | sugars: 5g | fiber: 5g | sodium: 523mg

Lemon Pepper Tilapia with Broccoli and Carrots

Prep time: 0 minutes | Cook time: 15 minutes | Serves 4

1 pound tilapia fillets	½ cup low-sodium vegetable broth
1 teaspoon lemon pepper seasoning	
	2 tablespoons fresh lemon juice
¼ teaspoon fine sea salt	1 pound broccoli crowns, cut into bite-size florets
2 tablespoons extra-virgin olive oil	
	8 ounces carrots, cut into ¼-inch thick rounds
2 garlic cloves, minced	
1 small yellow onion, sliced	

1. Sprinkle the tilapia fillets all over with the lemon pepper seasoning and salt. 2. Select the Sauté setting on the Instant Pot and heat the oil and garlic for 2 minutes, until the garlic is bubbling but not browned. Add the onion and sauté for about 3 minutes more, until it begins to soften. 3. Pour in the broth and lemon juice, then use a wooden spoon to nudge any browned bits from the bottom of the pot. Using tongs, add the fish fillets to the pot in a single layer; it's fine if they overlap slightly. Place the broccoli and carrots on top. 4. Secure the lid and set the Pressure Release to Sealing. Press the Cancel button to reset the cooking program, then select the Pressure Cook or Manual setting and set the cooking time for 1 minute at low pressure. (The pot will take about 10 minutes to come up to pressure before the cooking program begins.) 5. When the cooking program ends, let the pressure release naturally for 10 minutes (don't open the pot before the 10 minutes are up, even if the float valve has gone down), then move the Pressure Release to Venting to release any remaining steam. Open the pot. Use a fish spatula to transfer the vegetables and fillets to plates. Serve right away.

Per Serving:
calories: 243 | fat: 9g | protein: 28g | carbs: 15g | sugars: 4g | fiber: 5g | sodium: 348mg

Avo-Tuna with Croutons

Prep time: 10 minutes | Cook time: 0 minutes | Serves 3

2 (5-ounce) cans chunk-light tuna, drained	pepper
	3 avocados, halved and pitted
2 tablespoons low-fat mayonnaise	6 tablespoons packaged croutons
½ teaspoon freshly ground black	

1. In a medium bowl, combine the tuna, mayonnaise, and pepper, and mix well. 2. Top the avocados with the tuna mixture and croutons.

Per Serving:
calories: 441 | fat: 32g | protein: 23g | carbs: 22g | sugars: 2g | fiber: 14g | sodium: 284mg

Scallops and Asparagus Skillet

Prep time: 10 minutes | Cook time: 15 minutes | Serves 4

3 teaspoons extra-virgin olive oil, divided	¼ cup dry white wine
1 pound asparagus, trimmed and cut into 2-inch segments	Juice of 1 lemon
	2 garlic cloves, minced
1 tablespoon butter	¼ teaspoon freshly ground black pepper
1 pound sea scallops	

1. In a large skillet, heat 1½ teaspoons of oil over medium heat. 2. Add the asparagus and sauté for 5 to 6 minutes until just tender, stirring regularly. Remove from the skillet and cover with aluminum foil to keep warm. 3. Add the remaining 1½ teaspoons of oil and the butter to the skillet. When the butter is melted and sizzling, place the scallops in a single layer in the skillet. Cook for about 3 minutes on one side until nicely browned. Use tongs to gently loosen and flip the scallops, and cook on the other side for another 3 minutes until browned and cooked through. Remove and cover with foil to keep warm. 4. In the same skillet, combine the wine, lemon juice, garlic, and pepper. Bring to a simmer for 1 to 2 minutes, stirring to mix in any browned pieces left in the pan. 5. Return the asparagus and the cooked scallops to the skillet to coat with the sauce. Serve warm.

Per Serving:

calories: 252 | fat: 7g | protein: 26g | carbs: 15g | sugars: 3g | fiber: 2g | sodium: 493mg

Teriyaki Salmon

Prep time: 30 minutes | Cook time: 12 minutes | Serves 4

4 (6-ounce / 170-g) salmon fillets	¼ teaspoon ground ginger
	2 teaspoons olive oil
½ cup soy sauce	½ teaspoon salt
¼ cup packed light brown sugar	¼ teaspoon freshly ground black pepper
2 teaspoons rice vinegar	
1 teaspoon minced garlic	Oil, for spraying

1. Place the salmon in a small pan, skin-side up. 2. In a small bowl, whisk together the soy sauce, brown sugar, rice vinegar, garlic, ginger, olive oil, salt, and black pepper. 3. Pour the mixture over the salmon and marinate for about 30 minutes. 4. Line the air fryer basket with parchment and spray lightly with oil. Place the salmon in the prepared basket, skin-side down. You may need to work in batches, depending on the size of your air fryer. 5. Air fry at 400°F (204°C) for 6 minutes, brush the salmon with more marinade, and cook for another 6 minutes, or until the internal temperature reaches 145°F (63°C). Serve immediately.

Per Serving:

calories: 319 | fat: 14g | protein: 37g | carbs: 8g | sugars: 6g | fiber: 1g | sodium: 762mg

Baked Salmon with Lemon Sauce

Prep time: 10 minutes | Cook time: 15 minutes | Serves 4

4 (5-ounce) salmon fillets	Juice and zest of 1 lemon
Sea salt	1 teaspoon chopped fresh thyme
Freshly ground black pepper	½ cup fat-free sour cream
1 tablespoon extra-virgin olive oil	1 teaspoon honey
½ cup low-sodium vegetable broth	1 tablespoon chopped fresh chives

1. Preheat the oven to 400°F. 2. Season the salmon lightly on both sides with salt and pepper. 3. Place a large ovenproof skillet over medium-high heat and add the olive oil. 4. Sear the salmon fillets on both sides until golden, about 3 minutes per side. 5. Transfer the salmon to a baking dish and bake until it is just cooked through, about 10 minutes. 6. While the salmon is baking, whisk together the vegetable broth, lemon juice, zest, and thyme in a small saucepan over medium-high heat until the liquid reduces by about one-quarter, about 5 minutes. 7. Whisk in the sour cream and honey. 8. Stir in the chives and serve the sauce over the salmon.

Per Serving:

calories: 243 | fat: 10g | protein: 30g | carbs: 8g | sugars: 2g | fiber: 1g | sodium: 216mg

Greek Scampi

Prep time: 10 minutes | Cook time: 5 minutes | Serves 2

2 garlic cloves, minced	Juice of ½ lemon
2 tablespoons extra-virgin olive oil	2 teaspoons chopped fresh dill, or ¾ teaspoon dried
½ pound shrimp, peeled, deveined, and thoroughly rinsed	Dash salt
1 cup diced tomatoes	Dash freshly ground black pepper
½ cup nonfat ricotta cheese	Lemon wedges, for garnish
6 Kalamata olives	

1. In a large skillet set over medium heat, sauté the garlic in the olive oil for 30 seconds. 2. Add the shrimp. Cook for 1 minute. 3. Add the tomatoes, ricotta cheese, olives, lemon juice, and dill. Reduce the heat to low. Simmer for 5 to 10 minutes, stirring so the shrimp cook on both sides. When the shrimp are pink and the tomatoes and ricotta have made a sauce, the dish is ready. 4. Sprinkle with salt and pepper. 5. Serve immediately, garnished with lemon wedges.

Per Serving:

calories: 345 | fat: 21g | protein: 31g | carbs: 11g | sugars: 3g | fiber: 2g | sodium: 406mg

Shrimp with Tomatoes and Feta

Prep time: 10 minutes | Cook time: 30 minutes | Serves 4

3 tomatoes, coarsely chopped

½ cup chopped sun-dried tomatoes

2 teaspoons minced garlic

2 teaspoons extra-virgin olive oil

1 teaspoon chopped fresh oregano

Freshly ground black pepper

1½ pounds (16–20 count) shrimp, peeled, deveined, tails removed

4 teaspoons freshly squeezed lemon juice

½ cup low-sodium feta cheese, crumbled

1. Heat the oven to 450°F. 2. In a medium bowl, toss the tomatoes, sun-dried tomatoes, garlic, oil, and oregano until well combined. 3. Season the mixture lightly with pepper. 4. Transfer the tomato mixture to a 9-by-13-inch glass baking dish. 5. Bake until softened, about 15 minutes. 6. Stir the shrimp and lemon juice into the hot tomato mixture and top evenly with the feta. 7. Bake until the shrimp are cooked through, about 15 minutes more.

Per Serving:

calories: 252 | fat: 8g | protein: 39g | carbs: 9g | sugars: 6g | fiber: 2g | sodium: 396mg

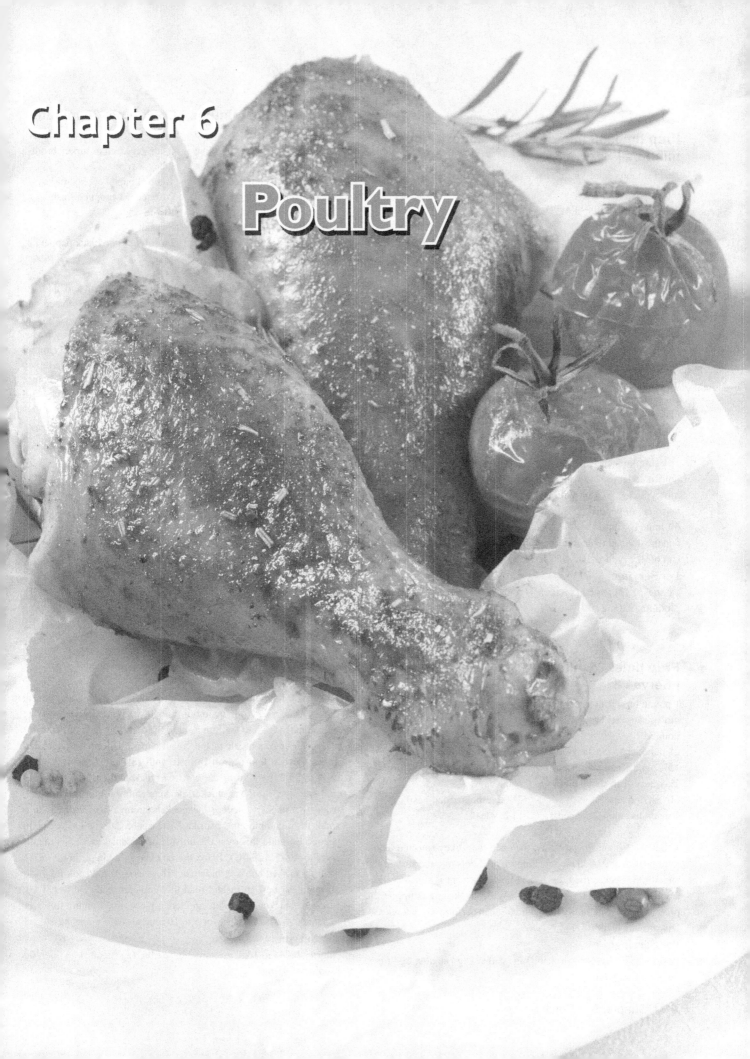

Chapter 6

Poultry

Mushroom-Sage Stuffed Turkey Breast

Prep time: 10 minutes | Cook time: 1 hour 5 minutes | Serves 8

2 tablespoons extra-virgin olive oil, divided
8 ounces brown mushrooms, finely chopped
2 garlic cloves, minced
½ teaspoon salt, divided
¼ teaspoon freshly ground black

pepper, divided
2 tablespoons chopped fresh sage
1 boneless, skinless turkey breast (about 3 pounds), butterflied

1. Preheat the oven to 375°F. 2. In a large skillet, heat 1 tablespoon of oil over medium heat. Add the mushrooms and cook for 4 to 5 minutes, stirring regularly, until most of the liquid has evaporated from the pan. Add the garlic, ¼ teaspoon of salt, and ⅛ teaspoon of pepper, and continue to cook for an additional minute. Add the sage to the pan, cook for 1 minute, and remove the pan from the heat. 3. On a clean work surface, lay the turkey breast flat. Use a kitchen mallet to pound the breast to an even 1-inch thickness throughout. 4. Spread the mushroom-sage mixture on the turkey breast, leaving a 1-inch border around the edges. Roll the breast tightly into a log. 5. Using kitchen twine, tie the breast two or three times around to hold it together. Rub the remaining 1 tablespoon of oil over the turkey breast. Season with the remaining ¼ teaspoon of salt and ⅛ teaspoon of pepper. 6. Transfer to a roasting pan and roast for 50 to 60 minutes, until the juices run clear, the meat is cooked through, and the internal temperature reaches 180°F. 7. Let rest for 5 minutes. Cut off the twine, slice, and serve.

Per Serving:
calories: 232 | fat: 6g | protein: 41g | carbs: 2g | sugars: 0g | fiber: 0g | sodium: 320mg

Pizza in a Pot

Prep time: 25 minutes | Cook time: 15 minutes | Serves 8

1 pound bulk lean sweet Italian turkey sausage, browned and drained
28 ounces can crushed tomatoes
15½ ounces can chili beans
2¼ ounces can sliced black olives, drained
1 medium onion, chopped

1 small green bell pepper, chopped
2 garlic cloves, minced
¼ cup grated Parmesan cheese
1 tablespoon quick-cooking tapioca
1 tablespoon dried basil
1 bay leaf

1. Set the Instant Pot to Sauté, then add the turkey sausage. Sauté until browned. 2. Add the remaining ingredients into the Instant Pot and stir. 3. Secure the lid and make sure the vent is set to sealing. Cook on Manual for 15 minutes. 4. When cook time is up, let the pressure release naturally for 5 minutes then perform a quick release. Discard bay leaf.

Per Serving:
calorie: 251 | fat: 10g | protein: 18g | carbs: 23g | sugars: 8g | fiber: 3g | sodium: 936mg

Turkey Cabbage Soup

Prep time: 15 minutes | Cook time: 30 minutes | Serves 4

1 tablespoon extra-virgin olive oil
1 sweet onion, chopped
2 celery stalks, chopped
2 teaspoons minced fresh garlic
4 cups finely shredded green cabbage
1 sweet potato, peeled, diced

8 cups chicken or turkey broth
2 bay leaves
1 cup chopped cooked turkey
2 teaspoons chopped fresh thyme
Sea salt
Freshly ground black pepper

1. Place a large saucepan over medium-high heat and add the olive oil. 2. Sauté the onion, celery, and garlic until softened and translucent, about 3 minutes. 3. Add the cabbage and sweet potato and sauté for 3 minutes. 4. Stir in the chicken broth and bay leaves and bring the soup to a boil. 5. Reduce the heat to low and simmer until the vegetables are tender, about 20 minutes. 6. Add the turkey and thyme and simmer until the turkey is heated through, about 4 minutes. 7. Remove the bay leaves and season the soup with salt and pepper.

Per Serving:
calorie: 444 | fat: 14g | protein: 38g | carbs: 46g | sugars: 17g | fiber: 7g | sodium: 427mg

Broccoli Cheese Chicken

Prep time: 10 minutes | Cook time: 19 to 24 minutes | Serves 6

1 tablespoon avocado oil
¼ cup chopped onion
½ cup finely chopped broccoli
4 ounces (113 g) cream cheese, at room temperature
2 ounces (57 g) Cheddar cheese, shredded
1 teaspoon garlic powder

½ teaspoon sea salt, plus additional for seasoning, divided
¼ freshly ground black pepper, plus additional for seasoning, divided
2 pounds (907 g) boneless, skinless chicken breasts
1 teaspoon smoked paprika

1. Heat a medium skillet over medium-high heat and pour in the avocado oil. Add the onion and broccoli and cook, stirring occasionally, for 5 to 8 minutes, until the onion is tender. 2. Transfer to a large bowl and stir in the cream cheese, Cheddar cheese, and garlic powder, and season to taste with salt and pepper. 3. Hold a sharp knife parallel to the chicken breast and cut a long pocket into one side. Stuff the chicken pockets with the broccoli mixture, using toothpicks to secure the pockets around the filling. 4. In a small dish, combine the paprika, ½ teaspoon salt, and ¼ teaspoon pepper. Sprinkle this over the outside of the chicken. 5. Set the air fryer to 400°F (204°C). Place the chicken in a single layer in the air fryer basket, cooking in batches if necessary, and cook for 14 to 16 minutes, until an instant-read thermometer reads 160°F (71°C). Place the chicken on a plate and tent a piece of aluminum foil over the chicken. Allow to rest for 5 to 10 minutes before serving.

Per Serving:
calorie: 287 | fat: 16g | protein: 32g | carbs: 1g | sugars: 0g | fiber: 0g | sodium: 291mg

Turkey Stuffed Peppers

Prep time: 15 minutes | Cook time: 50 minutes | Serves 4

1 teaspoon extra-virgin olive oil, plus more for greasing the baking dish	½ teaspoon chopped fresh basil
	Sea salt
	Freshly ground black pepper
1 pound ground turkey breast	4 red bell peppers, tops cut off, seeded
½ sweet onion, chopped	
1 teaspoon minced garlic	2 ounces low-sodium feta cheese
1 tomato, diced	

1. Preheat the oven to 350°F. 2. Lightly grease a 9-by-9-inch baking dish with olive oil and set it aside. 3. Place a large skillet over medium heat and add 1 teaspoon of olive oil. 4. Add the turkey to the skillet and cook until it is no longer pink, stirring occasionally to break up the meat and brown it evenly, about 6 minutes. 5. Add the onion and garlic and sauté until softened and translucent, about 3 minutes. 6. Stir in the tomato and basil. Season with salt and pepper. 7. Place the peppers cut-side up in the baking dish. Divide the filling into four equal portions and spoon it into the peppers. 8. Sprinkle the feta cheese on top of the filling. 9. Add ¼ cup of water to the dish and cover with aluminum foil. 10. Bake the peppers until they are soft and heated through, about 40 minutes.

Per Serving:
calorie: 285 | fat: 12g | protein: 31g | carbs: 12g | sugars: 8g | fiber: 3g | sodium: 79mg

BBQ Turkey Meat Loaf

Prep time: 5 minutes | Cook time: 40 minutes | Serves 6

1 pound 93 percent lean ground turkey	½ small yellow onion, finely diced
⅓ cup low-sugar or unsweetened barbecue sauce, plus 2 tablespoons	1 garlic clove, minced
	½ teaspoon fine sea salt
	½ teaspoon freshly ground black pepper
⅓ cup gluten-free panko (Japanese bread crumbs)	Cooked cauliflower "rice" or brown rice for serving
1 large egg	

1. Pour 1 cup water into the Instant Pot. Lightly grease a 7 by 3-inch round cake pan or a 5½ by 3-inch loaf pan with olive oil or coat with nonstick cooking spray. 2. In a medium bowl, combine the turkey, ⅓ cup barbecue sauce, panko, egg, onion, garlic, salt, and pepper and mix well with your hands until all of the ingredients are evenly distributed. Transfer the mixture to the prepared pan, pressing it into an even layer. Cover the pan tightly with aluminum foil. Place the pan on a long-handled silicone steam rack, then, holding the handles of the steam rack, lower it into the pot. (If you don't have the long-handled rack, use the wire metal steam rack and a homemade sling) 3. Secure the lid and set the Pressure Release to Sealing. Select the Pressure Cook or Manual setting and set the cooking time for 25 minutes at high pressure if using a 7-inch round cake pan, or for 35 minutes at high pressure if using a 5½ by 3-inch loaf pan. (The pot will take about 10 minutes to come up to pressure before the cooking program begins.) 4. Preheat a toaster oven or position an oven rack 4 to 6 inches below the heat source and preheat the broiler. 5. When the cooking program ends, perform a quick pressure release by moving the Pressure Release to Venting. Open the pot and, wearing heat-resistant mitts, grasp the handles of the steam rack and lift it out of the pot. Uncover the pan, taking care not to get burned by the steam or to drip condensation onto the meat loaf. Brush the remaining 2 tablespoons barbecue sauce on top of the meat loaf. 6. Broil the meat loaf for a few minutes, just until the glaze becomes bubbly and browned. Cut the meat loaf into slices and serve hot, with the cauliflower "rice" alongside.

Per Serving:
calories: 236 | fat: 11g | protein: 25g | carbs: 10g | sugars: 2g | fiber: 3g | sodium: 800mg

Easy Chicken Cacciatore

Prep time: 5 minutes | Cook time: 20 minutes | Serves 2

Extra-virgin olive oil cooking spray	chicken breasts, cubed
	1 cup sliced cremini mushrooms
1 garlic clove, chopped	½ cup chopped tomatoes, with juice
½ cup chopped red onion	
¾ cup chopped green bell pepper	1 cup green beans
	1 teaspoon dried oregano
2 (6-ounce) boneless skinless	1 teaspoon dried rosemary

1. Coat a skillet with cooking spray. Place it over medium heat. 2. Add the garlic. Sauté for about 1 minute, or until browned. 3. Add the red onion, green bell pepper, and chicken. Cook for about 6 minutes, or until the chicken is slightly browned, tossing to cook all sides. 4. Stir in the mushrooms, tomatoes, green beans, oregano, and rosemary. Reduce the heat to medium-low. Simmer for 8 to 10 minutes, stirring constantly. 5. Remove from the heat and serve hot. 6. Enjoy!

Per Serving:
calorie: 265 | fat: 5g | protein: 42g | carbs: 13g | sugars: 6g | fiber: 4g | sodium: 91mg

Greek Chicken

Prep time: 25 minutes | Cook time: 20 minutes | Serves 6

4 potatoes, unpeeled, quartered	3 teaspoons dried oregano
2 pounds chicken pieces, trimmed of skin and fat	¾ teaspoons salt
	½ teaspoons pepper
2 large onions, quartered	1 tablespoon olive oil
1 whole bulb garlic, cloves minced	1 cup water

1. Place potatoes, chicken, onions, and garlic into the inner pot of the Instant Pot, then sprinkle with seasonings. Top with oil and water. 2. Secure the lid and make sure vent is set to sealing. Cook on Manual mode for 20 minutes. 3. When cook time is over, let the pressure release naturally for 5 minutes, then release the rest manually.

Per Serving:
calorie: 278 | fat: 6g | protein: 27g | carbs: 29g | sugars: 9g | fiber: 4g | sodium: 358mg

Tantalizing Jerked Chicken

Prep time: 10 minutes | Cook time: 20 minutes | Serves 4

4 (5 ounces) boneless, skinless chicken breasts	1 tablespoon ground allspice
½ sweet onion, cut into chunks	2 teaspoons chopped fresh thyme
2 habanero chile peppers, halved lengthwise, seeded	1 teaspoon freshly ground black pepper
¼ cup freshly squeezed lime juice	½ teaspoon ground nutmeg
	¼ teaspoon ground cinnamon
2 tablespoons extra-virgin olive oil	2 cups fresh greens (such as arugula or spinach)
1 tablespoon minced garlic	1 cup halved cherry tomatoes

1. Place two chicken breasts in each of two large resealable plastic bags. Set them aside. 2. Place the onion, habaneros, lime juice, olive oil, garlic, allspice, thyme, black pepper, nutmeg, and cinnamon in a food processor and pulse until very well blended. 3. Pour half the marinade into each bag with the chicken breasts. Squeeze out as much air as possible, seal the bags, and place them in the refrigerator for 4 hours. 4. Preheat a barbecue to medium-high heat. 5. Let the chicken sit at room temperature for 15 minutes and then grill, turning at least once, until cooked through, about 15 minutes total. 6. Let the chicken rest for about 5 minutes before serving. Divide the greens and tomatoes among four serving plates, and top with the chicken.

Per Serving:

calorie: 268 | fat: 10g | protein: 33g | carbs: 9g | sugars: 4g | fiber: 2g | sodium: 74mg

Teriyaki Chicken and Broccoli

Prep time: 5 minutes | Cook time: 20 minutes | Serves 4

For The Sauce	For The Entrée
½ cup water	1 tablespoon sesame oil
2 tablespoons low-sodium soy sauce	4 (4 ounces) boneless, skinless chicken breasts, cut into bite-size cubes
2 tablespoons honey	
1 tablespoon rice vinegar	1 (12 ounces) bag frozen broccoli
¼ teaspoon garlic powder	
Pinch ground ginger	1 (12 ounces) bag frozen cauliflower rice
1 tablespoon cornstarch	

Make The Sauce: 1. In a small saucepan, whisk together the water, soy sauce, honey, rice vinegar, garlic powder, and ginger. Add the cornstarch and whisk until it is fully incorporated. 2. Over medium heat, bring the teriyaki sauce to a boil. Let the sauce boil for 1 minute to thicken. Remove the sauce from the heat and set aside. Make The Entrée 1. Heat a large skillet over medium-low heat. When hot, add the oil and the chicken. Cook for 5 to 7 minutes, until the chicken is cooked through, stirring as needed. 2. Steam the broccoli and cauliflower rice in the microwave according to the package instructions. 3. Divide the cauliflower rice into four equal portions. Put one-quarter of the broccoli and chicken over each portion and top with the teriyaki sauce.

Per Serving:

calorie: 256 | fat: 7g | protein: 30g | carbs: 20g | sugars: 11g | fiber: 4g | sodium: 347mg

Peach-Glazed Chicken over Dandelion Greens

Prep time: 10 minutes | Cook time: 30 minutes | Serves 4

4 boneless, skinless chicken thighs	Pinch ground cloves
	Pinch ground nutmeg
Juice of 1 lime	⅛ teaspoon vanilla extract
½ cup white vinegar	½ cup store-bought low-sodium chicken broth
2 garlic cloves, smashed	
1 cup frozen peaches	1 bunch dandelion greens, cut into ribbons
½ cup water	
Pinch ground cinnamon	1 medium onion, thinly sliced

1. Set oven to broil. In a bowl, combine the chicken, lime juice, vinegar, and garlic, coating the chicken thoroughly. 2. Meanwhile, to make the peach glaze, in a small pot, combine the peaches, water, cinnamon, cloves, nutmeg, and vanilla. Cook over medium heat, stirring often, for 10 minutes, or until the peaches have softened. 3. In a large cast iron skillet, bring the broth to a simmer over medium heat. 4. Add the greens, and sauté for 5 minutes, or until the greens are wilted. 5. Add the onion and cook, stirring occasionally, for 3 minutes, or until slightly reduced. 6. Add the chicken and cover with the peach glaze. 7. Transfer the pan to the oven, and broil for 10 to 12 minutes, or until the chicken is golden brown.

Per Serving:

calorie: 317 | fat: 9g | protein: 42g | carbs: 16g | sugars: 5g | fiber: 5g | sodium: 281mg

Baked Turkey Spaghetti

Prep time: 5 minutes | Cook time: 20 minutes | Serves 4

1 (10-ounce) package zucchini noodles	½ teaspoon dried oregano
	2 cups low-sodium spaghetti sauce
2 tablespoons extra-virgin olive oil, divided	
1 pound 93% lean ground turkey	½ cup shredded sharp Cheddar cheese

1. Pat zucchini noodles dry between two paper towels. 2. In an oven-safe medium skillet, heat 1 tablespoon of olive oil over medium heat. When hot, add the zucchini noodles. Cook for 3 minutes, stirring halfway through. 3. Add the remaining 1 tablespoon of oil, ground turkey, and oregano. Cook for 7 to 10 minutes, stirring and breaking apart, as needed. 4. Add the spaghetti sauce to the skillet and stir. 5. If your broiler is in the top of your oven, place the oven rack in the center position. Set the broiler on high. 6. Top the mixture with the cheese, and broil for 5 minutes or until the cheese is bubbly.

Per Serving:

calorie: 365 | fat: 23g | protein: 27g | carbs: 13g | sugars: 9g | fiber: 3g | sodium: 214mg

Grilled Lemon Mustard Chicken

Prep time: 5 minutes | Cook time: 15 minutes | Serves 6

Juice of 6 medium lemons	4 garlic cloves, minced
½ cup mustard seeds	2 tablespoons extra-virgin olive
1 tablespoon minced fresh	oil
tarragon	Three 8-ounce boneless,
2 tablespoons freshly ground	skinless chicken breasts, halved
black pepper	

1. In a small mixing bowl, combine the lemon juice, mustard seeds, tarragon, pepper, garlic, and oil; mix well. 2. Place the chicken in a baking dish, and pour the marinade on top. Cover, and refrigerate overnight. 3. Grill the chicken over medium heat for 10–15 minutes, basting with the marinade. Serve hot.

Per Serving:

calorie: 239 | fat: 11g | protein: 28g | carbs: 8g | sugars: 2g | fiber: 2g | sodium: 54mg

Pulled BBQ Chicken and Texas-Style Cabbage Slaw

Prep time: 5 minutes | Cook time: 20 minutes | Serves 6

Chicken	cut into narrow strips
1 cup water	2 carrots, julienned
¼ teaspoon fine sea salt	1 large Fuji or Gala apple,
3 garlic cloves, peeled	julienned
2 bay leaves	½ cup chopped fresh cilantro
2 pounds boneless, skinless	3 tablespoons fresh lime juice
chicken thighs (see Note)	3 tablespoons extra-virgin olive
Cabbage Slaw	oil
½ head red or green cabbage,	½ teaspoon ground cumin
thinly sliced	¼ teaspoon fine sea salt
1 red bell pepper, seeded and	¾ cup low-sugar or
thinly sliced	unsweetened barbecue sauce
2 jalapeño chiles, seeded and	Cornbread, for serving

1. To make the chicken: Combine the water, salt, garlic, bay leaves, and chicken thighs in the Instant Pot, arranging the chicken in a single layer. 2. Secure the lid and set the Pressure Release to Sealing. Select the Poultry, Pressure Cook, or Manual setting and set the cooking time for 10 minutes at high pressure. (The pot will take about 10 minutes to come up to pressure before the cooking program begins.) 3. To make the slaw: While the chicken is cooking, in a large bowl, combine the cabbage, bell pepper, jalapeños, carrots, apple, cilantro, lime juice, oil, cumin, and salt and toss together until the vegetables and apples are evenly coated. 4. When the cooking program ends, perform a quick pressure release by moving the Pressure Release to Venting, or let the pressure release naturally. Open the pot and, using tongs, transfer the chicken to a cutting board. Using two forks, shred the chicken into bite-size pieces. Wearing heat-resistant mitts, lift out the inner pot and discard the cooking liquid. Return the inner pot to the housing. 5. Return the chicken to the pot and stir in the barbecue sauce. You can serve it right away or heat it for a minute or

two on the Sauté setting, then return the pot to its Keep Warm setting until ready to serve. 6. Divide the chicken and slaw evenly among six plates. Serve with wedges of cornbread on the side.

Per Serving:

calories: 320 | fat: 14g | protein: 32g | carbs: 18g | sugars: 7g | fiber: 4g | sodium: 386mg

Jerk Chicken Casserole

Prep time: 15 minutes | Cook time: 45 minutes | Serves 6

1¼ teaspoons salt	1 can (15 ounces) black beans,
½ teaspoon pumpkin pie spice	drained, rinsed
¾ teaspoon ground allspice	1 large sweet potato (1 pound),
¾ teaspoon dried thyme leaves	peeled, cubed (3 cups)
¼ teaspoon ground red pepper	¼ cup honey
(cayenne)	¼ cup lime juice
6 boneless skinless chicken	2 teaspoons cornstarch
thighs	2 tablespoons sliced green
1 tablespoon vegetable oil	onions (2 medium)

1. Heat oven to 375°F. Spray 8-inch square (2-quart) glass baking dish with cooking spray. In small bowl, mix salt, pumpkin pie spice, allspice, thyme and red pepper. Rub mixture on all sides of chicken. In 12-inch nonstick skillet, heat oil over medium-high heat. Cook chicken in oil 2 to 3 minutes per side, until brown. 2. In baking dish, layer beans and sweet potato. Top with browned chicken. In small bowl, mix honey, lime juice and cornstarch; add to skillet. Heat to boiling, stirring constantly. Pour over chicken in baking dish. 3. Bake 35 to 45 minutes or until juice of chicken is clear when center of thickest part is cut (165°F) and sweet potatoes are fork-tender. Sprinkle with green onions.

Per Serving:

calories: 330 | fat: 8g | protein: 21g | carbs: 43g | sugars: 16g | fiber: 9g | sodium: 550mg

Chicken Provençal

Prep time: 5 minutes | Cook time: 25 minutes | Serves 4

2 tablespoons extra-virgin olive	½ cup dry white wine
oil	1 cup canned diced tomatoes
Two 8-ounce boneless, skinless	¼ cup pitted Kalamata olives
chicken breasts, halved	¼ cup finely chopped fresh basil
1 medium garlic clove, minced	⅛ teaspoon freshly ground black
¼ cup minced onion	pepper
¼ cup minced green bell pepper	

1. Heat the oil in a skillet over medium heat. Add the chicken, and brown about 3–5 minutes. 2. Add the remaining ingredients, and cook uncovered over medium heat for 20 minutes or until the chicken is no longer pink. Transfer to a serving platter and season with additional pepper to taste, if desired, before serving.

Per Serving:

calorie: 245 | fat: 11g | protein: 26g | carbs: 5g | sugars: 2g | fiber: 2g | sodium: 121mg

Roast Chicken with Pine Nuts and Fennel

Prep time: 20 minutes | Cook time: 30 minutes | Serves 2

For the herb paste
2 tablespoons fresh rosemary leaves
1 tablespoon freshly grated lemon zest
2 garlic cloves, quartered
½ teaspoon freshly ground black pepper
¼ teaspoon salt
1 teaspoon extra-virgin olive oil
For the chicken
4 (6-ounce) skinless chicken drumsticks

2 teaspoons extra-virgin olive oil
For the vegetables
1 large fennel bulb, cored and chopped (about 3 cups)
1 cup sliced fresh mushrooms
½ cup sliced carrots
¼ cup chopped sweet onion
2 teaspoons extra-virgin olive oil
2 tablespoons pine nuts
2 teaspoons white wine vinegar

To make the vegetables 1. Preheat the oven to 450°F. 2. In a 9-by-13-inch baking dish, toss together the fennel, mushrooms, carrots, onion, and olive oil. Place the dish in the preheated oven. Bake for 10 minutes. 3. Stir in the pine nuts. 4. Top with the browned drumsticks. Return the dish to the oven. Bake for 15 to 20 minutes more, or until the fennel is golden and an instant-read thermometer inserted into the thickest part of a drumstick without touching the bone registers 165°F. 5. Remove the chicken from the pan. 6. Stir the white wine vinegar into the pan. Toss the vegetables to coat, scraping up any browned bits. 7. Serve the chicken with the vegetables and enjoy!

Per Serving:
calorie: 316 | fat: 15g | protein: 35g | carbs: 10g | sugars: 4g | fiber: 3g | sodium: 384mg

Grilled Herb Chicken with Wine and Roasted Garlic

Prep time: 5 minutes | Cook time: 45 minutes | Serves 4

Four 3-ounce boneless, skinless chicken breast halves
2 tablespoons extra-virgin olive oil, divided
1 cup red wine
3 sprigs fresh thyme

5 garlic cloves, minced
5 garlic cloves, whole and unpeeled
⅛ teaspoon freshly ground black pepper

1. In a plastic zippered bag, place chicken, 1 tablespoon of the oil, wine, thyme, and minced garlic. Marinate for 2–3 hours in the refrigerator. 2. Preheat the oven to 375 degrees. 3. Spread the whole garlic cloves on a cookie sheet, drizzle with the remaining oil, and sprinkle with pepper. Bake for 30 minutes, stirring occasionally, until soft. 4. When cool, squeeze the garlic paste from the cloves, and mash in a small bowl with a fork. 5. Remove the chicken from the marinade, and grill for 12–15 minutes, turning frequently and brushing with garlic paste. Transfer to a platter, and serve hot.

Per Serving:

calorie: 222 | fat: 9g | protein: 20g | carbs: 4g | sugars: 0g | fiber: 0g | sodium: 40mg

Coconut Lime Chicken

Prep time: 5 minutes | Cook time: 15 minutes | Serves 4

1 tablespoon coconut oil
4 (4-ounce) boneless, skinless chicken breasts
½ teaspoon salt
1 red bell pepper, cut into ¼-inch-thick slices
16 asparagus spears, bottom ends trimmed

1 cup unsweetened coconut milk
2 tablespoons freshly squeezed lime juice
½ teaspoon garlic powder
¼ teaspoon red pepper flakes
¼ cup chopped fresh cilantro

1. In a large skillet, heat the oil over medium-low heat. When hot, add the chicken. 2. Season the chicken with the salt. Cook for 5 minutes, then flip. 3. Push the chicken to the side of the skillet, and add the bell pepper and asparagus. Cook, covered, for 5 minutes. 4. Meanwhile, in a small bowl, whisk together the coconut milk, lime juice, garlic powder, and red pepper flakes. 5. Add the coconut milk mixture to the skillet, and boil over high heat for 2 to 3 minutes. 6. Top with the cilantro.

Per Serving:
calorie: 319 | fat: 21g | protein: 28g | carbs: 7g | sugars: 4g | fiber: 2g | sodium: 353mg

Herbed Buttermilk Chicken

Prep time: 5 minutes | Cook time: 25 minutes | Serves 4

1½ pounds boneless, skinless chicken breasts
4 cups buttermilk
Pinch kosher salt
Pinch freshly ground black

pepper
1 cup thinly sliced yellow onion
2 tablespoons canola oil
¼ cup Italian seasoning
1 lemon, cut into wedges

1. In a large bowl or sealable plastic bag, combine the chicken, buttermilk, salt, and pepper. Cover or seal and refrigerate for at least 1 hour and up to 24 hours. 2. When the chicken is ready to cook, preheat the oven to 425°F. Line a baking sheet with parchment paper. 3. Remove the chicken from the buttermilk brine and pat it dry. Place the chicken on the prepared baking sheet along with the onion, and drizzle everything with the canola oil. Toss together on the baking sheet (this will save you a bowl) to coat the chicken and onion evenly. 4. Bake for 25 minutes or until the chicken is cooked through. (If the chicken is thick, you can cut the breasts in half lengthwise. It will cut down on your cook time by half or less. Check the chicken after it's cooked for 8 minutes if the breasts are thin.) 5. Allow the chicken to rest and sprinkle it and the onions with the Italian seasoning. 6. Serve with a squeeze of lemon juice.

Per Serving:
calorie: 380 | fat: 14g | protein: 47g | carbs: 16g | sugars: 13g | fiber: 1g | sodium: 543mg

Orange Chicken Thighs with Bell Peppers

Prep time: 15 to 20 minutes | Cook time: 7 minutes | Serves 4 to 6

6 boneless skinless chicken thighs, cut into bite-sized pieces	3 cloves garlic, minced or chopped
2 packets crystallized True Orange flavoring	½ teaspoon pink salt
½ teaspoon True Orange Orange Ginger seasoning	½ teaspoon black pepper
	1 teaspoon garlic powder
½ teaspoon coconut aminos	1 teaspoon ground ginger
¼ teaspoon Worcestershire sauce	¼ to ½ teaspoon red pepper flakes
Olive oil or cooking spray	2 tablespoons tomato paste
2 cups bell pepper strips, any color combination (I used red)	½ cup chicken bone broth or water
1 onion, chopped	1 tablespoon brown sugar substitute (I use Sukrin Gold)
1 tablespoon green onion, chopped fine	½ cup Seville orange spread (I use Crofter's brand)

1. Combine the chicken with the 2 packets of crystallized orange flavor, the orange ginger seasoning, the coconut aminos, and the Worcestershire sauce. Set aside. 2. Turn the Instant Pot to Sauté and add a touch of olive oil or cooking spray to the inner pot. Add in the orange ginger marinated chicken thighs. 3. Sauté until lightly browned. Add in the peppers, onion, green onion, garlic, and seasonings. Mix well. 4. Add the remaining ingredients; mix to combine. 5. Lock the lid, set the vent to sealing, set to 7 minutes. 6. Let the pressure release naturally for 2 minutes, then manually release the rest when cook time is up.

Per Serving:
calories: 120| fat: 2g | protein: 12g | carbs: 8g | sugars: 10g | fiber: 2g | sodium: 315mg

Chicken Caesar Salad

Prep time: 10 minutes | Cook time: 15 minutes | Serves 2

1 garlic clove	¼ teaspoon salt
½ teaspoon anchovy paste	Freshly ground black pepper
Juice of ½ lemon	2 romaine lettuce hearts, cored and chopped
2 tablespoons extra-virgin olive oil	1 red bell pepper, seeded and cut into thin strips
1 (8-ounce) boneless, skinless chicken breast	¼ cup grated Parmesan cheese

1. Preheat the broiler to high. 2. In a blender jar, combine the garlic, anchovy paste, lemon juice, and olive oil. Process until smooth and set aside. 3. Cut the chicken breast lengthwise into two even cutlets of similar thickness. Season the chicken with the salt and pepper, and place on a baking sheet. 4. Broil the chicken for 5 to 7 minutes on each side until cooked through and browned. Cut into thin strips. 5. In a medium mixing bowl, toss the lettuce, bell pepper, and cheese. Add the dressing and toss to coat. Divide the salad between 2 plates

and top with the chicken.

Per Serving:
calories: 292 | fat: 18g | protein: 28g | carbs: 6g | sugars: 3g | fiber: 2g | sodium: 706mg

Spice-Rubbed Turkey Breast

Prep time: 5 minutes | Cook time: 45 to 55 minutes | Serves 10

1 tablespoon sea salt	pepper
1 teaspoon paprika	4 pounds (1.8 kg) bone-in, skin-on turkey breast
1 teaspoon onion powder	
1 teaspoon garlic powder	2 tablespoons unsalted butter, melted
½ teaspoon freshly ground black	

1. In a small bowl, combine the salt, paprika, onion powder, garlic powder, and pepper. 2. Sprinkle the seasonings all over the turkey. Brush the turkey with some of the melted butter. 3. Set the air fryer to 350ºF (177ºC). Place the turkey in the air fryer basket, skin-side down, and roast for 25 minutes. 4. Flip the turkey and brush it with the remaining butter. Continue cooking for another 20 to 30 minutes, until an instant-read thermometer reads 160ºF (71ºC). 5. Remove the turkey breast from the air fryer. Tent a piece of aluminum foil over the turkey, and allow it to rest for about 5 minutes before serving.

Per Serving:
calorie: 331 | fat: 12g | protein: 49g | carbs: 2g | sugars: 0g | fiber: 1g | sodium: 2235mg

Herbed Whole Turkey Breast

Prep time: 10 minutes | Cook time:30 minutes | Serves 12

3 tablespoons extra-virgin olive oil	1 tablespoon kosher salt
1½ tablespoons herbes de Provence or poultry seasoning	1½ teaspoons freshly ground black pepper
2 teaspoons minced garlic	1 (6 pounds) bone-in, skin-on whole turkey breast, rinsed and patted dry
1 teaspoon lemon zest (from 1 small lemon)	

1. In a small bowl, whisk together the olive oil, herbes de Provence, garlic, lemon zest, salt, and pepper. 2. Rub the outside of the turkey and under the skin with the olive oil mixture. 3. Pour 1 cup of water into the electric pressure cooker and insert a wire rack or trivet. 4. Place the turkey on the rack, skin-side up. 5. Close and lock the lid of the pressure cooker. Set the valve to sealing. 6. Cook on high pressure for 30 minutes. 7. When the cooking is complete, hit Cancel. Allow the pressure to release naturally for 20 minutes, then quick release any remaining pressure. 8. Once the pin drops, unlock and remove the lid. 9. Carefully transfer the turkey to a cutting board. Remove the skin, slice, and serve.

Per Serving:
calorie: 389 | fat: 19g | protein: 50g | carbs: 1g | sugars: 0g | fiber: 0g | sodium: 582mg

Tangy Barbecue Strawberry-Peach Chicken

Prep time: 20 minutes | Cook time: 40 minutes | Serves 4

For the barbecue sauce	1 teaspoon garlic powder
1 cup frozen peaches	½ teaspoon cayenne pepper
1 cup frozen strawberries	½ teaspoon onion powder
¼ cup tomato purée	½ teaspoon freshly ground black
½ cup white vinegar	pepper
1 tablespoon yellow mustard	1 teaspoon celery seeds
1 teaspoon mustard seeds	For the chicken
1 teaspoon turmeric	4 boneless, skinless chicken
1 teaspoon sweet paprika	thighs

To make the barbecue sauce 1. In a stockpot, combine the peaches, strawberries, tomato purée, vinegar, mustard, mustard seeds, turmeric, paprika, garlic powder, cayenne, onion powder, black pepper, and celery seeds. Cook over low heat for 15 minutes, or until the flavors come together. 2. Remove the sauce from the heat, and let cool for 5 minutes. 3. Transfer the sauce to a blender, and purée until smooth. To make the chicken 1. Preheat the oven to 350°F. 2. Put the chicken in a medium bowl. Coat well with ½ cup of barbecue sauce. 3. Place the chicken on a rimmed baking sheet. 4. Place the baking sheet on the middle rack of the oven, and bake for about 20 minutes (depending on the thickness of thighs), or until the juices run clear. 5. Brush the chicken with additional sauce, return to the oven, and broil on high for 3 to 5 minutes, or until a light crust forms. 6. Serve.

Per Serving:

calorie: 389 | fat: 8g | protein: 63g | carbs: 13g | sugars: 7g | fiber: 3g | sodium: 175mg

Crispy Baked Drumsticks with Mustard Sauce

Prep time: 15 minutes | Cook time: 30 minutes | Serves 2

For The Chicken	4 (4-ounce) skinless chicken
Extra-virgin olive oil cooking	drumsticks, trimmed
spray	For The Mustard Sauce
⅓ cup almond meal	2 tablespoons plain nonfat
¼ teaspoon paprika	Greek yogurt
¼ teaspoon onion powder	1 tablespoon Dijon mustard
¼ teaspoon salt	¼ teaspoon liquid stevia
2 teaspoons extra-virgin olive	Freshly ground black pepper, to
oil	season
1 large egg	

Make The Chicken: 1. Preheat the oven to 475°F. 2. Coat a wire rack with cooking spray. Place the rack on a large rimmed baking sheet. 3. In a shallow dish, stir together the almond meal, paprika, onion powder, and salt. Drizzle with the olive oil. Mash together with a fork until the oil is thoroughly incorporated. 4. In another shallow dish, lightly beat the egg with a fork. 5. Working with 1 drumstick at a time, dip each into the egg, then press into the almond meal mixture, coating evenly on both sides. Place the chicken on the prepared rack. Repeat until all pieces are coated. 6. Place the sheet in the preheated oven. Bake for 25 to 30 minutes, or until golden and an instant-read thermometer inserted into the thickest part of a drumstick without touching the bone registers 165°F. Make The Mustard Sauce: 1. In a small bowl, stir together the yogurt, mustard, and stevia. Season with pepper. 2. Serve the sauce with the drumsticks.

Per Serving:

calorie: 423 | fat: 22g | protein: 51g | carbs: 5g | sugars: 2g | fiber: 2g | sodium: 425mg

Juicy Turkey Burgers

Prep time: 10 minutes | Cook time: 20 minutes | Serves 4

1½ pounds lean ground turkey	1 teaspoon chopped fresh thyme
½ cup bread crumbs	Sea salt
½ sweet onion, chopped	Freshly ground black pepper
1 carrot, peeled, grated	Nonstick cooking spray
1 teaspoon minced garlic	

1. In a large bowl, mix together the turkey, bread crumbs, onion, carrot, garlic, and thyme until very well mixed. 2. Season the mixture lightly with salt and pepper. 3. Shape the turkey mixture into 4 equal patties. 4. Place a large skillet over medium-high heat and coat it lightly with cooking spray. 5. Cook the turkey patties until golden and completely cooked through, about 10 minutes per side. 6. Serve the burgers plain or with your favorite toppings on a whole-wheat bun.

Per Serving:

calorie: 330 | fat: 15g | protein: 34g | carbs: 15g | sugars: 4g | fiber: 1g | sodium: 230mg

Chicken with Spiced Sesame Sauce

Prep time: 20 minutes | Cook time: 8 minutes | Serves 5

2 tablespoons tahini (sesame	1 teaspoon red wine vinegar
sauce)	2 teaspoons minced garlic
¼ cup water	1 teaspoon shredded ginger root
1 tablespoon low-sodium soy	(Microplane works best)
sauce	2 pounds chicken breast,
¼ cup chopped onion	chopped into 8 portions

1. Place first seven ingredients in bottom of the inner pot of the Instant Pot. 2. Add coarsely chopped chicken on top. 3. Secure the lid and make sure vent is at sealing. Set for 8 minutes using Manual setting. When cook time is up, let the pressure release naturally for 10 minutes, then perform a quick release. 4. Remove ingredients and shred chicken with fork. Combine with other ingredients in pot for a tasty sandwich filling or sauce.

Per Serving:

calorie: 215 | fat: 7g | protein: 35g | carbs: 2g | sugars: 0g | fiber: 0g | sodium: 178mg

Turkey Bolognese with Chickpea Pasta

Prep time: 5 minutes | Cook time: 25 minutes | Serves 4

1 onion, coarsely chopped	1 pound ground turkey
1 large carrot, coarsely chopped	½ cup milk
2 celery stalks, coarsely chopped	¾ cup red or white wine
1 tablespoon extra-virgin olive oil	1 (28-ounce) can diced tomatoes
	10 ounces cooked chickpea pasta

1. Place the onion, carrots, and celery in a food processor and pulse until finely chopped. 2. Heat the extra-virgin olive oil in a Dutch oven or medium skillet over medium-high heat. Sauté the chopped vegetables for 3 to 5 minutes, or until softened. Add the ground turkey, breaking the poultry into smaller pieces, and cook for 5 minutes. 3. Add the milk and wine and cook until the liquid is nearly evaporated (turn up the heat to high to quicken the process). 4. Add the tomatoes and bring the sauce to a simmer. Reduce the heat to low and simmer for 10 to 15 minutes. 5. Meanwhile, cook the pasta according to the package instructions and set aside. 6. Serve the sauce with the cooked chickpea pasta. 7. Store any leftovers in an airtight container in the refrigerator for 3 to 4 days.

Per Serving:
calorie: 419 | fat: 15g | protein: 31g | carbs: 34g | sugars: 8g | fiber: 11g | sodium: 150mg

Sesame-Ginger Chicken Soba

Prep time: 10 minutes | Cook time: 15 minutes | Serves 6

8 ounces soba noodles	1 (1-inch) piece fresh ginger, finely grated
2 boneless, skinless chicken breasts, halved lengthwise	⅓ cup water
¼ cup tahini	1 large cucumber, seeded and diced
2 tablespoons rice vinegar	1 scallions bunch, green parts only, cut into 1-inch segments
1 tablespoon reduced-sodium gluten-free soy sauce or tamari	1 tablespoon sesame seeds
1 teaspoon toasted sesame oil	

1. Preheat the broiler to high. 2. Bring a large pot of water to a boil. Add the noodles and cook until tender, according to the package directions. Drain and rinse the noodles in cool water. 3. On a baking sheet, arrange the chicken in a single layer. Broil for 5 to 7 minutes on each side, depending on the thickness, until the chicken is cooked through and its juices run clear. Use two forks to shred the chicken. 4. In a small bowl, combine the tahini, rice vinegar, soy sauce, sesame oil, ginger, and water. Whisk to combine. 5. In a large bowl, toss the shredded chicken, noodles, cucumber, and scallions. Pour the tahini sauce over the noodles and toss to combine. Served sprinkled with the sesame seeds.

Per Serving:
calories: 251 | fat: 8g | protein: 16g | carbs: 35g | sugars: 2g | fiber: 2g | sodium: 482mg

Shredded Buffalo Chicken

Prep time: 10 minutes | Cook time: 20 minutes | Serves 8

2 tablespoons avocado oil	½ tablespoon apple cider vinegar
½ cup finely chopped onion	¼ teaspoon garlic powder
1 celery stalk, finely chopped	2 bone-in, skin-on chicken breasts (about 2 pounds)
1 large carrot, chopped	
⅓ cup mild hot sauce (such as Frank's RedHot)	

1. Set the electric pressure cooker to the Sauté setting. When the pot is hot, pour in the avocado oil. 2. Sauté the onion, celery, and carrot for 3 to 5 minutes or until the onion begins to soften. Hit Cancel. 3. Stir in the hot sauce, vinegar, and garlic powder. Place the chicken breasts in the sauce, meat-side down. 4. Close and lock the lid of the pressure cooker. Set the valve to sealing. 5. Cook on high pressure for 20 minutes. 6. When cooking is complete, hit Cancel and quick release the pressure. Once the pin drops, unlock and remove the lid. 7. Using tongs, transfer the chicken breasts to a cutting board. When the chicken is cool enough to handle, remove the skin, shred the chicken and return it to the pot. Let the chicken soak in the sauce for at least 5 minutes. 8. Serve immediately.

Per Serving:
calorie: 235 | fat: 14g | protein: 24g | carbs: 2g | sugars: 1g | fiber: 1g | sodium: 142mg

Turkey with Almond Duxelles

Prep time: 5 minutes | Cook time:35 minutes | Serves 8

2 tablespoons extra-virgin olive oil	½ cup ground almonds
¼ cup dry sherry	¼ teaspoon freshly ground black pepper
¾ pound diced fresh mushrooms	2 pounds turkey breast cutlets, pounded to ¼-inch thickness and cut into 8 portions
4 medium shallots, finely minced	
2 garlic cloves, minced	Paprika, for garnish
1 teaspoon minced fresh thyme	½ cup low-fat plain Greek yogurt
Dash cayenne pepper	

1. Preheat the oven to 350 degrees. 2. In a large skillet over medium heat, heat the olive oil and sherry. Add the mushrooms, shallots, garlic, thyme, and cayenne pepper. Cook, stirring often, until the mushrooms turn dark. Add the ground almonds, dash salt (optional), and pepper, and sauté for 2–3 minutes. 3. Divide the mixture into 8 portions, and place each portion in the center of each turkey portion. Fold the edges over, roll up, and place in a baking dish, seam side down, 1 inch apart. 4. Place about 1 tablespoon Greek yogurt over each turkey roll, and sprinkle with paprika. Bake at 350 degrees for 25–30 minutes or until the turkey is tender. Transfer to a serving platter, and serve.

Per Serving:
calorie: 216 | fat: 9g | protein: 30g | carbs: 5g | sugars: 2g | fiber: 1g | sodium: 97mg

Buttermilk-Ginger Smothered Chicken

Prep time: 30 minutes | Cook time: 20 minutes | Serves 8

8 boneless, skinless chicken thighs	½ bunch fresh cilantro, thinly sliced
2 cups low-fat buttermilk	2 garlic cloves, minced
½ bunch fresh chives, thinly sliced	1 teaspoon ground ginger

1. Preheat the oven to 375°F. 2. In a large bowl, combine the chicken, buttermilk, chives, cilantro, garlic, and ginger, coating the chicken thoroughly. Cover and put in the refrigerator to marinate for at least 30 minutes. 3. Place the chicken in a Dutch oven and cover. Transfer to the oven and cook for 20 minutes, or until the chicken is moist on the inside and caramelized on the outside. 4. Serve.

Per Serving:
calorie: 363 | fat: 8g | protein: 64g | carbs: 4g | sugars: 3g | fiber: 0g | sodium: 188mg

Chicken in Wine

Prep time: 10 minutes | Cook time: 12 minutes | Serves 6

2 pounds chicken breasts, trimmed of skin and fat	10¾-ounce can French onion soup
10¾-ounce can 98% fat-free, reduced-sodium cream of mushroom soup	1 cup dry white wine or chicken broth

1. Place the chicken into the Instant Pot. 2. Combine soups and wine. Pour over chicken. 3. Secure the lid and make sure vent is set to sealing. Cook on Manual mode for 12 minutes. 4. When cook time is up, let the pressure release naturally for 5 minutes and then release the rest manually.

Per Serving:
calories: 225 | fat: 5g | protein: 35g | carbs: 7g | sugars: 3g | fiber: 1g | sodium: 645mg

Smothered Dijon Chicken

Prep time: 10 minutes | Cook time: 30 minutes | Serves 4

¾ cup low-fat buttermilk	2 boneless, skinless chicken breasts
2 tablespoons Dijon mustard	
3 garlic cloves, minced	2 large carrots, peeled and halved
1 tablespoon dried dill	
1 teaspoon mustard seeds	1 medium onion, quartered

1. Preheat the oven to 375°F. 2. In a medium bowl, combine the buttermilk, mustard, garlic, dill, and mustard seeds. Mix well. 3. Add the chicken, carrots, and onion, coating them thoroughly with the buttermilk mixture. Set aside to marinate for at least 15 minutes. 4. Place the chicken, carrots, and onions on a rimmed baking sheet. Discard the remaining buttermilk mixture. 5. Transfer the baking sheet to the oven, and bake for 30 minutes, or until the vegetables are tender, and the chicken is cooked through and its juices run clear. Serve warm and enjoy.

Per Serving:
calorie: 223 | fat: 5g | protein: 34g | carbs: 10g | sugars: 5g | fiber: 2g | sodium: 261mg

Creamy Nutmeg Chicken

Prep time: 20 minutes | Cook time: 10 minutes | Serves 6

1 tablespoon canola oil	mushroom soup
6 boneless chicken breast halves, skin and visible fat removed	½ cup fat-free sour cream
	½ cup fat-free milk
¼ cup chopped onion	1 tablespoon ground nutmeg
¼ cup minced parsley	¼ teaspoon sage
2 (10¾-ounce) cans 98% fat-free, reduced-sodium cream of	¼ teaspoon dried thyme
	¼ teaspoon crushed rosemary

1. Press the Sauté button on the Instant Pot and then add the canola oil. Place the chicken in the oil and brown chicken on both sides. Remove the chicken to a plate. 2. Sauté the onion and parsley in the remaining oil in the Instant Pot until the onions are tender. Press Cancel on the Instant Pot, then place the chicken back inside. 3. Mix together the remaining ingredients in a bowl then pour over the chicken. 4. Secure the lid and set the vent to sealing. Set on Manual mode for 10 minutes. 5. When cooking time is up, let the pressure release naturally.

Per Serving:
calories: 264 | fat: 8g | protein: 31g | carbs: 15g | sugars: 5g | fiber: 1g | sodium: 495mg

Orange Chicken

Prep time: 10 minutes | Cook time: 10 minutes | Serves 4

3 tablespoons extra-virgin olive oil	Juice and zest of 1 orange
	1 teaspoon cornstarch
1 pound chicken breasts or thighs, cut into ¾-inch pieces	½ teaspoon sriracha (or to taste)
	Sesame seeds (optional, for garnish)
1 teaspoon peeled and grated fresh ginger	
	Thinly sliced scallion (optional, for garnish)
2 garlic cloves, minced	
1 tablespoon honey	

1. In a large skillet over medium-high heat, heat the olive oil until it shimmers. Add the chicken to the oil and cook, stirring occasionally, until opaque, about 5 minutes. Add the ginger and garlic and cook, stirring constantly, for 30 seconds. 2. In a small bowl, whisk together the honey, orange juice and zest, cornstarch, and sriracha. Add the sauce mixture to the chicken and cook, stirring, until the sauce thickens, about 2 minutes. 3. Serve garnished with sesame seeds and sliced scallions, if desired.

Per Serving:
calorie: 264 | fat: 15g | protein: 23g | carbs: 10g | sugars: 8g | fiber: 1g | sodium: 109mg

Italian Chicken Thighs

Prep time: 5 minutes | Cook time: 20 minutes | Serves 2

4 bone-in, skin-on chicken thighs

2 tablespoons unsalted butter, melted

1 teaspoon dried parsley

1 teaspoon dried basil

½ teaspoon garlic powder

¼ teaspoon onion powder

¼ teaspoon dried oregano

1. Brush chicken thighs with butter and sprinkle remaining ingredients over thighs. Place thighs into the air fryer basket. 2. Adjust the temperature to 380ºF (193ºC) and roast for 20 minutes. 3. Halfway through the cooking time, flip the thighs. 4. When fully cooked, internal temperature will be at least 165ºF (74ºC) and skin will be crispy. Serve warm.

Per Serving:

calorie: 446 | fat: 34g | protein: 33g | carbs: 2g | sugars: 0g | fiber: 0g | sodium: 163mg

Grain-Free Parmesan Chicken

Prep time: 5 minutes | Cook time: 20 minutes | Serves 4

1½ cups (144 g) almond flour

½ cup (50 g) grated Parmesan cheese

1 tablespoon (3 g) Italian seasoning

1 teaspoon garlic powder

½ teaspoon black pepper

2 large eggs

4 (6 ounces [170 g], ½-inch [13 mm]-thick) boneless, skinless chicken breasts

½ cup (120 ml) no-added-sugar marinara sauce

½ cup (56 g) shredded mozzarella cheese

2 tablespoons (8 g) minced fresh herbs of choice (optional)

1. Preheat the oven to 375°F (191°C). Line a large, rimmed baking sheet with parchment paper. 2. In a shallow dish, mix together the almond flour, Parmesan cheese, Italian seasoning, garlic powder, and black pepper. In another shallow dish, whisk the eggs. Dip a chicken breast into the egg wash, then gently shake off any extra egg. Dip the chicken breast into the almond flour mixture, coating it well. Place the chicken breast on the prepared baking sheet. Repeat this process with the remaining chicken breasts. 3. Bake the chicken for 15 to 20 minutes, or until the meat is no longer pink in the center. 4. Remove the chicken from the oven and flip each breast. Top each breast with 2 tablespoons (30 ml) of marinara sauce and 2 tablespoons (14 g) of mozzarella cheese. 5. Increase the oven temperature to broil and place the chicken back in the oven. Broil it until the cheese is melted and just starting to brown. Carefully remove the chicken from the oven, top it with the herbs (if using), and let it rest for about 10 minutes before serving.

Per Serving:

calorie: 572 | fat: 32g | protein: 60g | carbs: 13g | sugars: 4g | fiber:5g | sodium: 560mg

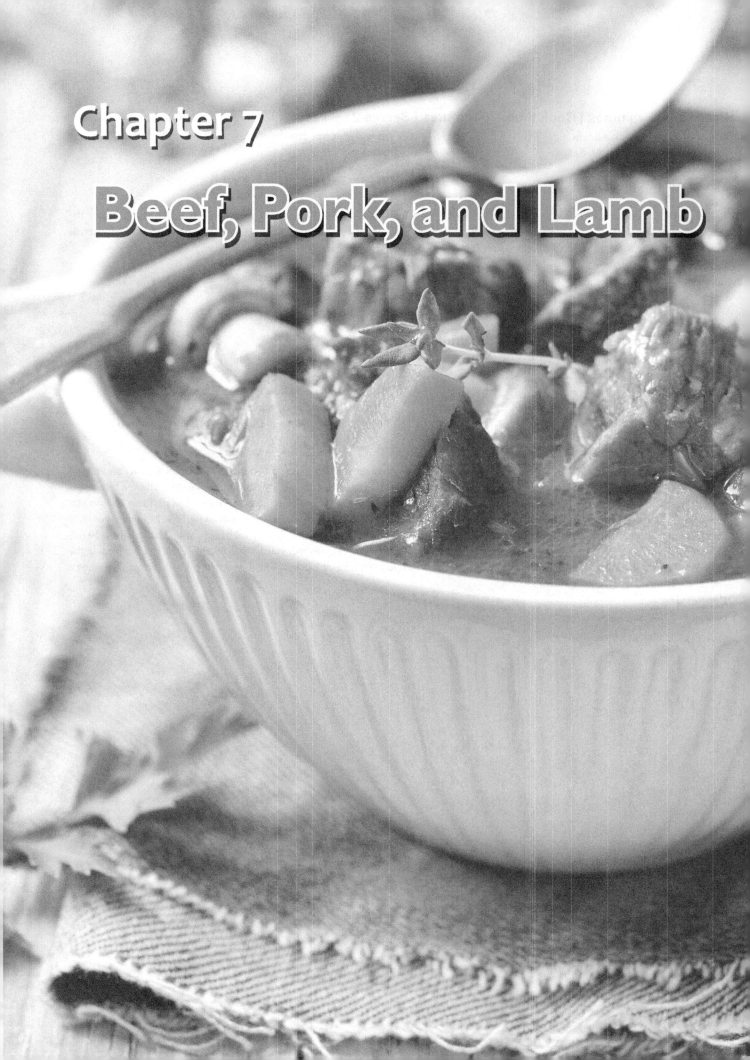

Chapter 7
Beef, Pork, and Lamb

Beef Burrito Bowl

Prep time: 5 minutes | Cook time: 15 minutes | Serves 4

1 pound 93% lean ground beef	¼ teaspoon salt
1 cup canned low-sodium black beans, drained and rinsed	1 head romaine or preferred lettuce, shredded
¼ teaspoon ground cumin	2 medium tomatoes, chopped
¼ teaspoon chili powder	1 cup shredded Cheddar cheese or packaged cheese blend
¼ teaspoon garlic powder	
¼ teaspoon onion powder	

1. Heat a large skillet over medium-low heat. Put the beef, beans, cumin, chili powder, garlic powder, onion powder, and salt into the skillet, and cook for 8 to 10 minutes, until cooked through. Stir occasionally. 2. Divide the lettuce evenly between four bowls. Add one-quarter of the beef mixture to each bowl and top with one-quarter of the tomatoes and cheese.

Per Serving:

caloric: 358 | fat. 16g | protein: 37g | carbs: 18g | sugars: 4g | fiber: 8g | sodium: 506mg

Shepherd's Pie with Cauliflower-Carrot Mash

Prep time: 10 minutes | Cook time: 35 minutes | Serves 6

1 tablespoon coconut oil	sauce
2 garlic cloves, minced	One 12-ounce bag frozen baby lima beans, green peas, or shelled edamame
1 large yellow onion, diced	
1 pound ground lamb	3 tablespoons tomato paste
1 pound 95 percent lean ground beef	1 pound cauliflower florets
½ cup low-sodium vegetable broth	1 pound carrots, halved lengthwise and then crosswise (or quartered if very large)
1 teaspoons dried thyme	
1 teaspoon dried sage	¼ cup coconut milk or other nondairy milk
1 teaspoon freshly ground black pepper	½ cup sliced green onions, white and green parts
1¾ teaspoons fine sea salt	
2 tablespoons Worcestershire	

1. Select the Sauté setting on the Instant Pot and heat the oil and garlic for 2 minutes, until the garlic is bubbling but not browned. Add the onion and sauté for 3 minutes, until it begins to soften. Add the lamb and beef and sauté, using a wooden spoon or spatula to break up the meat as it cooks, for 6 minutes, until cooked through and no streaks of pink remain. 2. Stir in the broth, using the spoon or spatula to nudge any browned bits from the bottom of the pot. Add the thyme, sage, pepper, ¾ teaspoon of the salt, the Worcestershire sauce, and lima beans and stir to mix. Dollop the tomato paste on top. Do not stir it in. 3. Place a tall steam rack in the pot, then place the cauliflower and carrots on top of the rack. 4. Secure the lid and set the Pressure Release to Sealing. Press the Cancel button to reset the cooking program, then select the Pressure Cook or Manual setting and set the cooking time for 4 minutes at low pressure. (The pot will take about 15 minutes to come up to pressure before the cooking program begins.) 5. Position an oven rack 4 to 6 inches below the heat source and preheat the broiler. 6. When the cooking program ends, perform a quick pressure release by moving the Pressure Release to Venting. Open the pot and, using tongs, transfer the cauliflower and carrots to a bowl. Add the coconut milk and remaining 1 teaspoon salt to the bowl. Using an immersion blender, blend the vegetables until smooth. 7. Wearing heat-resistant mitts, remove the steam rack from the pot. Stir ½ cup of the mashed vegetables into the filling mixture in the pot, incorporating the tomato paste at the same time. Remove the inner pot from the housing. Transfer the mixture to a broiler-safe 9 by 13-inch baking dish, spreading it in an even layer. Dollop the mashed vegetables on top and spread them out evenly with a fork. Broil, checking often, for 5 to 8 minutes, until the mashed vegetables are lightly browned. 8. Spoon the shepherd's pie onto plates, sprinkle with the green onions, and serve hot.

Per Serving:

calories: 437 | fat: 18g | protein: 39g | carbs: 33g | sugars: 8g | fiber: 9g | sodium: 802mg

Spicy Beef Stew with Butternut Squash

Prep time: 15 minutes | Cook time: 30 minutes | Serves 8

1½ tablespoons smoked paprika	1 cup low-sodium beef or vegetable broth
2 teaspoons ground cinnamon	
1½ teaspoons kosher salt	1 medium red onion, cut into wedges
1 teaspoon ground ginger	
1 teaspoon red pepper flakes	8 garlic cloves, minced
½ teaspoon freshly ground black pepper	1 (28-ounce) carton or can no-salt-added diced tomatoes
2 pounds beef shoulder roast, cut into 1-inch cubes	2 pounds butternut squash, peeled and cut into 1-inch pieces
2 tablespoons avocado oil, divided	Chopped fresh cilantro or parsley, for serving

1. In a zip-top bag or medium bowl, combine the paprika, cinnamon, salt, ginger, red pepper, and black pepper. Add the beef and toss to coat. 2. Set the electric pressure cooker to the Sauté setting. When the pot is hot, pour in 1 tablespoon of avocado oil. 3. Add half of the beef to the pot and cook, stirring occasionally, for 3 to 5 minutes or until the beef is no longer pink. Transfer it to a plate, then add the remaining 1 tablespoon of avocado oil and brown the remaining beef. Transfer to the plate. Hit Cancel. 4. Stir in the broth and scrape up any brown bits from the bottom of the pot. Return the beef to the pot and add the onion, garlic, tomatoes and their juices, and squash. Stir well. 5. Close and lock lid of pressure cooker. Set the valve to sealing. 6. Cook on high pressure for 30 minutes. 7. When cooking is complete, hit Cancel. Allow the pressure to release naturally for 10 minutes, then quick release any remaining pressure. 8. Unlock and remove lid. 9. Spoon into serving bowls, sprinkle with cilantro or parsley, and serve.

Per Serving:

calorie: 275 | fat: 9g | protein: 28g | carbs: 24g | sugars: 7g | fiber: 6g | sodium: 512mg

Easy Beef Curry

Prep time: 15 minutes | Cook time: 10 minutes | Serves 6

1 tablespoon extra-virgin olive oil	through
1 small onion, thinly sliced	¼ teaspoon ground turmeric
2 teaspoons minced fresh ginger	¼ teaspoon salt
3 garlic cloves, minced	1 pound grass-fed sirloin tip
2 teaspoons ground coriander	steak, top round steak, or top
1 teaspoon ground cumin	sirloin steak, cut into bite-size
1 jalapeño or serrano pepper, slit	pieces
lengthwise but not all the way	2 tablespoons chopped fresh
	cilantro

1. In a large skillet, heat the oil over medium high. 2. Add the onion, and cook for 3 to 5 minutes until browned and softened. Add the ginger and garlic, stirring continuously until fragrant, about 30 seconds. 3. In a small bowl, mix the coriander, cumin, jalapeño, turmeric, and salt. Add the spice mixture to the skillet and stir continuously for 1 minute. Deglaze the skillet with about ¼ cup of water. 4. Add the beef and stir continuously for about 5 minutes until well-browned yet still medium rare. Remove the jalapeño. Serve topped with the cilantro.

Per Serving:

calories: 140 | fat: 7g | protein: 18g | carbs: 3g | sugars: 1g | fiber: 1g | sodium: 141mg

Red Wine Pot Roast with Winter Vegetables

Prep time: 10 minutes | Cook time: 1 hour 35 minutes | Serves 6

One 3-pound boneless beef chuck roast or bottom round roast (see Note)	1 cup dry red wine
	2 tablespoons Dijon mustard
2 teaspoons fine sea salt	2 teaspoons chopped fresh rosemary
1 teaspoon freshly ground black pepper	1 pound parsnips or turnips, cut into ½-inch pieces
1 tablespoon cold-pressed avocado oil	1 pound carrots, cut into ½-inch pieces
4 large shallots, quartered	4 celery stalks, cut into ½-inch
4 garlic cloves, minced	pieces

1. Put the beef onto a plate, pat it dry with paper towels, and then season all over with the salt and pepper. 2. Select the Sauté setting on the Instant Pot and heat the oil for 2 minutes. Using tongs, lower the roast into the pot and sear for about 4 minutes, until browned on the first side. Flip the roast and sear for about 4 minutes more, until browned on the second side. Return the roast to the plate. 3. Add the shallots to the pot and sauté for about 2 minutes, until they begin to soften. Add the garlic and sauté for about 1 minute more. Stir in the wine, mustard, and rosemary, using a wooden spoon to nudge any browned bits from the bottom of the pot. Return the roast to the pot, then spoon some of the cooking liquid over the top. 4. Secure the lid and set the Pressure Release to Sealing. Press the Cancel button to reset the cooking program, then select the Meat/Stew setting and set the cooking time for 1 hour 5 minutes at high pressure. (The pot will take about 5 minutes to come up to pressure before the cooking program begins.) 5. When the cooking program ends, let the pressure release naturally for at least 15 minutes, then move the Pressure Release to Venting to release any remaining steam. Open the pot and, using tongs, carefully transfer the pot roast to a cutting board. Tent with aluminum foil to keep warm. 6. Add the parsnips, carrots, and celery to the pot. 7. Secure the lid and set the Pressure Release to Sealing. Press the Cancel button to reset the cooking program, then select the Pressure Cook or Manual setting and set the cooking time for 3 minutes at low pressure. (The pot will take about 10 minutes to come up to pressure before the cooking program begins.) 8. When the cooking program ends, perform a quick pressure release by moving the Pressure Release to Venting. Open the pot and, using a slotted spoon, transfer the vegetables to a serving dish. Wearing heat-resistant mitts, lift out the inner pot and pour the cooking liquid into a gravy boat or other serving vessel with a spout. (If you like, use a fat separator to remove the fat from the liquid before serving.) 9. If the roast was tied, snip the string and discard. Carve the roast against the grain into ½-inch-thick slices and arrange them on the dish with the vegetables. Pour some cooking liquid over the roast and serve, passing the remaining cooking liquid on the side.

Per Serving:

calorie: 448 | fat: 25g | protein: 26g | carbs: 26g | sugars: 7g | fiber: 6g | sodium: 945mg

Mango-Glazed Pork Tenderloin Roast

Prep time: 10 minutes | Cook time: 20 minutes | Serves 4

1 pound boneless pork tenderloin, trimmed of fat	1 teaspoon extra-virgin olive oil
	1 tablespoon honey
1 teaspoon chopped fresh rosemary	2 tablespoons white wine vinegar
1 teaspoon chopped fresh thyme	2 tablespoons dry cooking wine
¼ teaspoon salt, divided	1 tablespoon minced fresh
¼ teaspoon freshly ground black pepper, divided	ginger
	1 cup diced mango

1. Preheat the oven to 400°F. 2. Season the tenderloin with the rosemary, thyme, ⅛ teaspoon of salt, and ⅛ teaspoon of pepper. 3. Heat the olive oil in an oven-safe skillet over medium-high heat, and sear the tenderloin until browned on all sides, about 5 minutes total. 4. Transfer the skillet to the oven and roast for 12 to 15 minutes until the pork is cooked through, the juices run clear, and the internal temperature reaches 145°F. Transfer to a cutting board to rest for 5 minutes. 5. In a small bowl, combine the honey, vinegar, cooking wine, and ginger. In to the same skillet, pour the honey mixture and simmer for 1 minute. Add the mango and toss to coat. Transfer to a blender and purée until smooth. Season with the remaining ⅛ teaspoon of salt and ⅛ teaspoon of pepper. 6. Slice the pork into rounds and serve with the mango sauce.

Per Serving:

calories: 182 | fat: 4g | protein: 24 | carbs: 12g | sugars: 10g | fiber: 1g | sodium: 240mg

Bacon and Cheese Stuffed Pork Chops

Prep time: 10 minutes | Cook time: 12 minutes | Serves 4

½ ounce (14 g) plain pork rinds, finely crushed	bacon, crumbled
½ cup shredded sharp Cheddar cheese	4 (4-ounce / 113-g) boneless pork chops
4 slices cooked sugar-free	½ teaspoon salt
	¼ teaspoon ground black pepper

1. In a small bowl, mix pork rinds, Cheddar, and bacon. 2. Make a 3-inch slit in the side of each pork chop and stuff with ¼ pork rind mixture. Sprinkle each side of pork chops with salt and pepper. 3. Place pork chops into ungreased air fryer basket, stuffed side up. Adjust the temperature to 400°F (204°C) and air fry for 12 minutes. Pork chops will be browned and have an internal temperature of at least 145°F (63°C) when done. Serve warm.

Per Serving:
calorie: 366 | fat: 16g | protein: 51g | carbs: 0g | sugars: 0g | fiber: 0g | sodium: 531mg

Pork Tacos

Prep time: 30 minutes | Cook time: 10 minutes | Serves 2

8 ounces boneless skinless pork tenderloin, thinly sliced, ¼-inch thick, across the grain	juice
Pinch salt	2 (6-inch) soft low-carb corn tortillas, such as La Tortilla
⅓ cup ancho chile sauce	4 tablespoons diced tomatoes, divided
2 tablespoons chipotle purée (see Recipe Tip)	1 cup shredded lettuce, divided
¼ cup freshly squeezed lime	½ avocado, sliced
	4 tablespoons salsa, divided

1. Sprinkle the pork slices with salt. Set aside. 2. In a small bowl, stir together the ancho chile sauce, chipotle purée, and lime juice. Reserve 3 tablespoons of the marinade. Set aside. 3. In a large sealable plastic bag, add the pork. Pour the remaining marinade over it. Seal the bag, removing as much air as possible. Marinate the meat for 20 minutes to 1 hour at room temperature, or refrigerate for several hours. Turn the meat twice while it marinates. 4. Place a small nonstick skillet over medium heat. Have a large piece of aluminum foil nearby. 5. Working with one tortilla at a time, heat both sides in the skillet until they puff slightly. As they are done, stack the tortillas on the foil. When they are all heated, wrap the tortillas in the foil. 6. Preheat the broiler. 7. Adjust the rack so it is 4 inches from the heating element. 8. Remove the pork slices from the marinade. Discard the marinade. Place the pork on a rack set over a sheet pan. 9. Place the pan in the oven. Broil for 3 to 4 minutes, or until the edges of the pork begin to brown. Remove from the oven. Turn and brush the pork with the reserved marinade. Broil the second side for 3 minutes, or until the pork is just barely pink inside. 10. Place the foil packet with the tortillas in the oven to warm while the pork finishes cooking. 11. To serve, pile each tortilla with a few slices of pork. Top each with about 2 tablespoons of diced tomato, ½ cup of shredded lettuce, half of the avocado slices, and about 2 tablespoons of salsa.

Per Serving:
calorie: 328 | fat: 13g | protein: 30g | carbs: 25g | sugars: 5g | fiber: 7g | sodium: 563mg

Pork Chop Diane

Prep time: 10 minutes | Cook time: 20 minutes | Serves 4

¼ cup low-sodium chicken broth	loin chops, about 1 inch thick
1 tablespoon freshly squeezed lemon juice	Sea salt
2 teaspoons Worcestershire sauce	Freshly ground black pepper
2 teaspoons Dijon mustard	1 teaspoon extra-virgin olive oil
4 (5-ounce) boneless pork top	1 teaspoon lemon zest
	1 teaspoon butter
	2 teaspoons chopped fresh chives

1. In a small bowl, stir together the chicken broth, lemon juice, Worcestershire sauce, and Dijon mustard and set it aside. 2. Season the pork chops lightly with salt and pepper. 3. Place a large skillet over medium-high heat and add the olive oil. 4. Cook the pork chops, turning once, until they are no longer pink, about 8 minutes per side. 5. Transfer the chops to a plate and set it aside. 6. Pour the broth mixture into the skillet and cook until warmed through and thickened, about 2 minutes. 7. Whisk in the lemon zest, butter, and chives. 8. Serve the chops with a generous spoonful of sauce.

Per Serving:
calorie: 203 | fat: 7g | protein: 32g | carbs: 1g | sugars: 0g | fiber: 0g | sodium: 130mg

Marinated Leg of Lamb

Prep time: 5 minutes | Cook time: 40 minutes | Serves 16

1 leg of lamb (7 pounds including bone), boned, butterflied, and visible fat removed	1 large carrot, thinly sliced
	6 parsley sprigs
	2 bay leaves, crumbled
3 cups dry red wine	4 cloves garlic, minced
¼ cup extra-virgin olive oil	⅛ teaspoon freshly ground black pepper
2 medium onions, sliced	Fresh parsley sprigs

1. In a large ceramic, glass, or stainless steel dish (anything but plastic), combine all the ingredients except the parsley sprigs; cover, refrigerate, and let marinate for 1–2 days, turning occasionally. 2. After marinating, drain the lamb, discard the marinade, and pat dry. Season with salt, if desired. Place the lamb into a grill basket. Broil the lamb 3–4 inches from the heat for 15–20 minutes per side. 3. Transfer the lamb to a cutting board and let cool slightly. Carve the lamb diagonally; transfer to a serving platter, garnish with parsley sprigs, and serve.

Per Serving:
calorie: 326 | fat: 13g | protein: 42g | carbs: 3g | sugars: 1g | fiber: 1g | sodium: 131mg

Teriyaki Rib-Eye Steaks

Prep time: 10 minutes | Cook time: 15 minutes | Serves 2

2 tablespoons water	¼ teaspoon garlic powder
1 tablespoon reduced-sodium soy sauce	⅛ teaspoon ground
1½ teaspoons Worcestershire sauce	2 (6 ounces) lean beef rib-eye steaks
1¼ teaspoons distilled white vinegar	Extra-virgin olive oil cooking spray
1 teaspoon extra-virgin olive oil	2 cups sugar snap peas
½ teaspoon granulated stevia	1 cup sliced carrots
½ teaspoon onion powder	1 red bell pepper, sliced

1. In a large bowl, whisk together the water, soy sauce, Worcestershire sauce, white vinegar, olive oil, stevia, onion powder, garlic powder, and ginger. 2. With a fork, pierce the steaks several times. Add to the marinade. Let marinate in the refrigerator for at least 2 hours. 3. Spray a large skillet with cooking spray. Place it over medium heat. 4. Add the steaks. Cook for 7 minutes. Turn the steaks. Add the sugar snap peas, carrots, and bell pepper to the skillet. Cook for 7 minutes more, or until an instant-read thermometer inserted into the center of the steak reads 140°F. 5. Serve and savor!

Per Serving:

calorie: 630 | fat: 40g | protein: 40g | carbs: 29g | sugars: 12g | fiber: 9g | sodium: 271mg

30-Minute Garlic Lamb Lollipops

Prep time: 10 minutes | Cook time: 10 minutes | Serves 4

2 tablespoons (18 g) minced garlic	½ teaspoon sea salt
¼ cup (60 ml) avocado or olive oil	¼ teaspoon black pepper
	12 to 16 ounces (340 to 454 g) lamb rib chops
2 tablespoons (30 ml) red wine vinegar	1 tablespoon (15 ml) avocado or grapeseed oil
1 tablespoon (3 g) Italian seasoning	Minced fresh rosemary, thyme, or basil, as needed

1. In a small bowl, combine the garlic, avocado oil, vinegar, Italian seasoning, salt, and black pepper. Whisk to mix the ingredients. 2. Place the lamb rib chops in an airtight container, like a plastic bag or glass storage container. Pour the marinade over the lamb rib chops and let them marinate at room temperature for 10 to 15 minutes. 3. Heat the avocado or grapeseed oil in a large cast-iron skillet over medium-high heat. Gently add the lamb rib chops to the skillet and cook them for 4 minutes. Flip the lamb and cook the meat for another 4 minutes, until it is brown on both sides. 4. Remove lamb rib chops from the skillet, and let them rest for 10 minutes before serving. Garnish them with the herbs and serve.

Per Serving:

calorie: 568 | fat: 55g | protein: 19g | carbs: 2g | sugars: 0g | fiber: 0g | sodium: 361mg

Italian Sausages with Peppers and Onions

Prep time: 5 minutes | Cook time: 28 minutes | Serves 3

1 medium onion, thinly sliced	coconut oil
1 yellow or orange bell pepper, thinly sliced	1 teaspoon fine sea salt
1 red bell pepper, thinly sliced	6 Italian sausages
¼ cup avocado oil or melted	Dijon mustard, for serving (optional)

1. Preheat the air fryer to 400°F (204°C). 2. Place the onion and peppers in a large bowl. Drizzle with the oil and toss well to coat the veggies. Season with the salt. 3. Place the onion and peppers in a pie pan and cook in the air fryer for 8 minutes, stirring halfway through. Remove from the air fryer and set aside. 4. Spray the air fryer basket with avocado oil. Place the sausages in the air fryer basket and air fry for 20 minutes, or until crispy and golden brown. During the last minute or two of cooking, add the onion and peppers to the basket with the sausages to warm them through. 5. Place the onion and peppers on a serving platter and arrange the sausages on top. Serve Dijon mustard on the side, if desired. 6. Store leftovers in an airtight container in the fridge for up to 7 days or in the freezer for up to a month. Reheat in a preheated 390°F (199°C) air fryer for 3 minutes, or until heated through.

Per Serving:

calorie: 455 | fat: 33g | protein: 29g | carbs: 13g | sugars: 3g | fiber: 2g | sodium: 392mg

Bavarian Beef

Prep time: 35 minutes | Cook time: 1 hour 15 minutes | Serves 8

1 tablespoon canola oil	broth
3-pound boneless beef chuck roast, trimmed of fat	⅓ cup German-style mustard
3 cups sliced carrots	2 teaspoons coarsely ground black pepper
3 cups sliced onions	2 bay leaves
2 large kosher dill pickles, chopped	¼ teaspoon ground cloves
1 cup sliced celery	1 cup water
½ cup dry red wine or beef	⅓ cup flour

1. Press Sauté on the Instant Pot and add in the oil. Brown roast on both sides for about 5 minutes. Press Cancel. 2. Add all of the remaining ingredients, except for the flour, to the Instant Pot. 3. Secure the lid and make sure the vent is set to sealing. Press Manual and set the time to 1 hour and 15 minutes. Let the pressure release naturally. 4. Remove meat and vegetables to large platter. Cover to keep warm. 5. Remove 1 cup of the liquid from the Instant Pot and mix with the flour. Press Sauté on the Instant Pot and add the flour/broth mixture back in, whisking. Cook until the broth is smooth and thickened. 6. Serve over noodles or spaetzle.

Per Serving:

calories: 251 | fat: 8g | protein: 26g | carbs: 17g | sugars: 7g | fiber: 4g | sodium: 525mg

Marjoram-Pepper Steaks

Prep time: 5 minutes | Cook time: 8 minutes | Serves 2

1 tablespoon freshly ground black pepper	1 tablespoon extra-virgin olive oil
¼ teaspoon dried marjoram	¼ cup low-sodium beef broth
2 (6-ounce, 1-inch-thick) beef tenderloins	Fresh marjoram sprigs, for garnish

1. In a large bowl, mix together the pepper and marjoram. 2. Add the steaks. Coat both sides with the spice mixture. 3. In a skillet set over medium-high heat, heat the olive oil. 4. Add the steaks. Cook for 5 to 7 minutes, or until an instant-read thermometer inserted in the center registers 160°F (for medium). Remove from the skillet. Cover to keep warm. 5. Add the broth to the skillet. Increase the heat to high. Bring to a boil, scraping any browned bits from the bottom. Boil for about 1 minute, or until the liquid is reduced by half. 6. Spoon the broth sauce over the steaks. Garnish with marjoram sprigs and serve immediately.

Per Serving:

calorie: 339 | fat: 19g | protein: 38g | carbs: 2g | sugars: 0g | fiber: 1g | sodium: 209mg

BBQ Ribs and Broccoli Slaw

Prep time: 10 minutes | Cook time: 50 minutes | Serves 6

BBQ Ribs	1 pound broccoli florets (or florets from 2 large crowns), chopped
4 pounds baby back ribs	
1 teaspoon fine sea salt	
1 teaspoon freshly ground black pepper	10 radishes, halved and thinly sliced
Broccoli Slaw	1 red bell pepper, seeded and cut lengthwise into narrow strips
½ cup plain 2 percent Greek yogurt	
1 tablespoon olive oil	1 large apple (such as Fuji, Jonagold, or Gala), thinly sliced
1 tablespoon fresh lemon juice	
½ teaspoon fine sea salt	½ red onion, thinly sliced
¼ teaspoon freshly ground black pepper	¾ cup low-sugar or unsweetened barbecue sauce

1. To make the ribs: Pat the ribs dry with paper towels, then cut the racks into six sections (three to five ribs per section, depending on how big the racks are). Season the ribs all over with the salt and pepper. 2. Pour 1 cup water into the Instant Pot and place the wire metal steam rack into the pot. Place the ribs on top of the wire rack (it's fine to stack them up). 3. Secure the lid and set the Pressure Release to Sealing. Select the Pressure Cook or Manual setting and set the cooking time for 20 minutes at high pressure. (The pot will take about 15 minutes to come up to pressure before the cooking program begins.) 4. To make the broccoli slaw: While the ribs are cooking, in a small bowl, stir together the yogurt, oil, lemon juice, salt, and pepper, mixing well. In a large bowl, combine the broccoli, radishes, bell pepper, apple, and onion. Drizzle with the yogurt mixture and toss until evenly coated. 5. When the ribs have about 10 minutes left in their cooking time, preheat the oven to 400°F. Line a sheet pan with aluminum foil. 6. When the cooking program ends, perform a quick pressure release by moving the Pressure Release to Venting. Open the pot and, using tongs, transfer the ribs in a single layer to the prepared sheet pan. Brush the barbecue sauce onto both sides of the ribs, using 2 tablespoons of sauce per section of ribs. Bake, meaty-side up, for 15 to 20 minutes, until lightly browned. 7. Serve the ribs warm, with the slaw on the side.

Per Serving:

calories: 392 | fat: 15g | protein: 45g | carbs: 19g | sugars: 9g | fiber: 4g | sodium: 961mg

Flank Steak with Smoky Honey Mustard Sauce

Prep time: 30 minutes | Cook time: 17 to 20 minutes | Serves 6

Sauce	(from 7 ounces can), finely chopped
¼ cup fat-free honey mustard or honey Dijon dressing	
	Steak
1 tablespoon frozen (thawed) orange juice concentrate	1 beef flank steak (about 1½ pounds)
1 tablespoon water	6 flour tortillas for burritos (8 inch), heated as directed on package
1 clove garlic, finely chopped	
1 chipotle chile in adobo sauce	

1. Heat gas or charcoal grill. In small bowl, mix sauce ingredients. On both sides of beef, make cuts about ½ inch apart and 1/8 inch deep in diamond pattern. Brush 2 tablespoons of the sauce on both sides of beef. 2 . Place beef on grill over medium heat. Cover grill; cook 17 to 20 minutes, turning once, until beef is of desired doneness. 3. Cut beef across grain into thin slices. Serve with tortillas and remaining sauce.

Per Serving:

calories: 310 | fat: 9g | protein: 36g | carbs: 22g | sugars: 2g | fiber: 0g | sodium: 380mg

Easy Pot Roast and Vegetables

Prep time: 20 minutes | Cook time: 35 minutes | Serves 6

3–4 pound chuck roast, trimmed of fat and cut into serving-sized chunks	4 medium carrots, sliced, or 1 pound baby carrots
	2 celery ribs, sliced thin
4 medium potatoes, cubed, unpeeled	1 envelope dry onion soup mix
	3 cups water

1. Place the pot roast chunks and vegetables into the Instant Pot along with the potatoes, carrots and celery. 2. Mix together the onion soup mix and water and pour over the contents of the Instant Pot. 3. Secure the lid and make sure the vent is set to sealing. Set the Instant Pot to Manual mode for 35 minutes. Let pressure release naturally when cook time is up.

Per Serving:

calorie: 325 | fat: 8g | protein: 35g | carbs: 26g | sugars: 6g | fiber: 4g | sodium: 560mg

Spinach and Provolone Steak Rolls

Prep time: 10 minutes | Cook time: 12 minutes | Makes 8 rolls

1 (1 pound / 454 g) flank steak, butterflied	1 cup fresh spinach leaves
8 (1 ounce / 28 g, ¼-inch-thick) deli slices provolone cheese	½ teaspoon salt
	¼ teaspoon ground black pepper

1. Place steak on a large plate. Place provolone slices to cover steak, leaving 1-inch at the edges. Lay spinach leaves over cheese. Gently roll steak and tie with kitchen twine or secure with toothpicks. Carefully slice into eight pieces. Sprinkle each with salt and pepper. 2. Place rolls into ungreased air fryer basket, cut side up. Adjust the temperature to 400ºF (204ºC) and air fry for 12 minutes. Steak rolls will be browned and cheese will be melted when done and have an internal temperature of at least 150ºF (66ºC) for medium steak and 180ºF (82ºC) for well-done steak. Serve warm.

Per Serving:

calorie: 155 | fat: 8g | protein: 19g | carbs: 1g | sugars: 0g | fiber: 0g | sodium: 351mg

Smothered Sirloin

Prep time: 15 minutes | Cook time: 30 minutes | Serves 5

1 pound beef round sirloin tip	2 celery stalks, thinly sliced
1 teaspoon freshly ground black pepper	1 medium red bell pepper, chopped
1 teaspoon celery seeds	2 garlic cloves, minced
2 tablespoons extra-virgin olive oil	2 tablespoons whole-wheat flour
1 medium yellow onion, chopped	Generous pinch cayenne pepper
¼ cup chickpea flour	Chopped fresh chives, for garnish (optional)
2 cups store-bought low-sodium chicken broth, divided	Smoked paprika, for garnish (optional)

1. In a bowl, season the steak on both sides with the black pepper and celery seeds. 2. Select the Sauté setting on an electric pressure cooker, and combine the olive oil and onions. Cook for 3 to 5 minutes, stirring, or until the onions are browned but not burned. 3. Slowly add the chickpea flour, 1 tablespoon at a time, while stirring. 4. Add 1 cup of broth, ¼ cup at a time, as needed. 5. Stir in the celery, bell pepper, and garlic and cook for 3 to 5 minutes, or until softened. 6. Lay the beef on top of vegetables, and pour the remaining 1 cup of broth on top. 7. Close and lock the lid and set the pressure valve to sealing. 8. Change to the Manual/Pressure Cook setting, and cook for 20 minutes. 9. Once cooking is complete, quick-release the pressure. Carefully remove the lid. 10. Remove the steak and vegetables from the pressure cooker, reserving the leftover liquid for the gravy base. 11. To make the gravy, add the whole-wheat flour and cayenne to the liquid in the pressure cooker, mixing continuously until thickened. 12. To serve, spoon the gravy over the steak and garnish with the chives (if using) and paprika (if using).

Per Serving:

calorie: 234 | fat: 11g | protein: 23g | carbs: 11g | sugars: 3g | fiber: 2g | sodium: 96mg

Creole Steak

Prep time: 5 minutes | Cook time: 1 hour 40 minutes | Serves 4

2 teaspoons extra-virgin olive oil	¼ teaspoon celery seed
¼ cup chopped onion	4 cloves garlic, finely chopped
¼ cup chopped green bell pepper	¼ teaspoon salt
1 cup canned crushed tomatoes	1 teaspoon cumin
½ teaspoon chili powder	1 pound lean boneless round steak

1. In a large skillet over medium heat, heat the oil. Add the onions and green pepper, and sauté until the onions are translucent (about 5 minutes). 2. Add the tomatoes, chili powder, celery seed, garlic, salt, and cumin; cover and let simmer over low heat for 20–25 minutes. This allows the flavors to blend. 3. Preheat the oven to 350 degrees. Trim all visible fat off the steak. 4. In a nonstick pan or a pan that has been sprayed with nonstick cooking spray, lightly brown the steak on each side. Transfer the steak to a 13-x-9-x-2-inch baking dish; pour the sauce over the steak, and cover. 5. Bake for 1¼ hours or until the steak is tender. Remove from the oven; slice the steak, and arrange on a serving platter. Spoon the sauce over the steak, and serve.

Per Serving:

calorie: 213 | fat: 10g | protein: 25g | carbs: 5g | sugars: 2g | fiber: 2g | sodium: 235mg

Beef Roast with Onions and Potatoes

Prep time: 30 minutes | Cook time: 9 to 10 hours | Serves 6

1 large sweet onion, cut in half, then cut into thin slices	to 2-inch cubes
1 boneless beef bottom round roast (3 lb), trimmed of excess fat	2 cloves garlic, finely chopped
	1¾ cups beef-flavored broth
	1 package (1 oz) onion soup mix (from 2-oz box)
3 baking potatoes, cut into 1½-	¼ cup all-purpose flour

1. Spray 5- to 6-quart slow cooker with cooking spray. In slow cooker, place onion. If beef roast comes in netting or is tied, remove netting or strings. Place beef on onion. Place potatoes and garlic around beef. In small bowl, mix 1¼ cups of the broth and the dry soup mix; pour over beef. (Refrigerate remaining broth.) 2. Cover; cook on Low heat setting 9 to 10 hours. 3. Remove beef and vegetables from slow cooker; place on serving platter. Cover to keep warm. 4. In small bowl, mix remaining ½ cup broth and the flour; gradually stir into juices in slow cooker. Increase heat setting to High. Cover; cook about 15 minutes, stirring occasionally, until sauce has thickened. Serve sauce over beef and vegetables.

Per Serving:

calorie: 416 | fat: 9g | protein: 54g | carbs: 27g | sugars: 4g | fiber: 3g | sodium: 428mg

Steaks with Walnut-Blue Cheese Butter

Prep time: 30 minutes | Cook time: 10 minutes | Serves 6

½ cup unsalted butter, at room temperature	1 teaspoon minced garlic
½ cup crumbled blue cheese	¼ teaspoon cayenne pepper
2 tablespoons finely chopped walnuts	Sea salt and freshly ground black pepper, to taste
1 tablespoon minced fresh rosemary	1½ pounds (680 g) New York strip steaks, at room temperature

1. In a medium bowl, combine the butter, blue cheese, walnuts, rosemary, garlic, and cayenne pepper and salt and black pepper to taste. Use clean hands to ensure that everything is well combined. Place the mixture on a sheet of parchment paper and form it into a log. Wrap it tightly in plastic wrap. Refrigerate for at least 2 hours or freeze for 30 minutes. 2. Season the steaks generously with salt and pepper. 3. Place the air fryer basket or grill pan in the air fryer. Set the air fryer to 400ºF (204ºC) and let it preheat for 5 minutes. 4. Place the steaks in the basket in a single layer and air fry for 5 minutes. Flip the steaks, and cook for 5 minutes more, until an instant-read thermometer reads 120ºF (49ºC) for medium-rare (or as desired). 5. Transfer the steaks to a plate. Cut the butter into pieces and place the desired amount on top of the steaks. Tent a piece of aluminum foil over the steaks and allow to sit for 10 minutes before serving. 6. Store any remaining butter in a sealed container in the refrigerator for up to 2 weeks.

Per Serving:

calorie: 620 | fat: 56g | protein: 26g | carbs: 2g | sugars: 0g | fiber: 1g | sodium: 442mg

Jalapeño Popper Pork Chops

Prep time: 15 minutes | Cook time: 6 to 8 minutes | Serves 4

1¾ pounds (794 g) bone-in, center-cut loin pork chops	4 ounces (113 g) sliced bacon, cooked and crumbled
Sea salt and freshly ground black pepper, to taste	4 ounces (113 g) Cheddar cheese, shredded
6 ounces (170 g) cream cheese, at room temperature	1 jalapeño, seeded and diced
	1 teaspoon garlic powder

1. Cut a pocket into each pork chop, lengthwise along the side, making sure not to cut it all the way through. Season the outside of the chops with salt and pepper. 2. In a small bowl, combine the cream cheese, bacon, Cheddar cheese, jalapeño, and garlic powder. Divide this mixture among the pork chops, stuffing it into the pocket of each chop. 3. Set the air fryer to 400ºF (204ºC). Place the pork chops in the air fryer basket in a single layer, working in batches if necessary. Air fry for 3 minutes. Flip the chops and cook for 3 to 5 minutes more, until an instant-read thermometer reads 145ºF (63ºC). 4. Allow the chops to rest for 5 minutes, then serve warm.

Per Serving:

calorie: 469 | fat: 21g | protein: 60g | carbs: 5g | sugars: 3g | fiber: 0g | sodium: 576mg

Sirloin Steaks with Cilantro Chimichurri

Prep time: 25 minutes | Cook time: 7 to 10 minutes | Serves 4

1 cup loosely packed fresh cilantro	2 teaspoons canola oil
1 small onion, cut into quarters	½ teaspoon salt
2 cloves garlic, cut in half	2 teaspoons ground cumin
1 jalapeño chile, cut in half, seeded	½ teaspoon pepper
2 teaspoons lime juice	4 beef sirloin steaks, 1 inch thick (about 1½ pound)

1. Heat gas or charcoal grill. In food processor, place cilantro, onion, garlic, chile, lime juice, oil and ¼ teaspoon of the salt. Cover; process until finely chopped. Blend in 2 to 3 teaspoons water to make sauce thinner, if desired. Transfer to small bowl; set aside until serving time. 2. In small bowl, mix cumin, pepper and remaining ¼ teaspoon salt; rub evenly over steaks. Place steaks on grill over medium heat. Cover grill; cook 7 to 10 minutes for medium-rare (145°F), turning once halfway through cooking. 3. Serve 2 tablespoons chimichurri over each steak.

Per Serving:

calorie: 266 | fat: 10g | protein: 38g | carbs: 3g | sugars: 1g | fiber: 1g | sodium: 392mg

Zoodles Carbonara

Prep time: 10 minutes | Cook time: 25 minutes | Serves 4

6 slices bacon, cut into pieces	3 large eggs, beaten
1 red onion, finely chopped	1 tablespoon heavy cream
3 zucchini, cut into noodles	Pinch red pepper flakes
1 cup peas	½ cup grated Parmesan cheese (optional, for garnish)
½ teaspoon sea salt	
3 garlic cloves, minced	

1. In a large skillet over medium-high heat, cook the bacon until browned, about 5 minutes. With a slotted spoon, transfer the bacon to a plate. 2. Add the onion to the bacon fat in the pan and cook, stirring, until soft, 3 to 5 minutes. Add the zucchini, peas, and salt. Cook, stirring, until the zucchini softens, about 3 minutes. Add the garlic and cook, stirring constantly, for 5 minutes. 3. In a small bowl, whisk together the eggs, cream, and red pepper flakes. Add to the vegetables. 4. Remove the pan from the stove top and stir for 3 minutes, allowing the heat of the pan to cook the eggs without setting them. 5. Return the bacon to the pan and stir to mix. 6. Serve topped with Parmesan cheese, if desired.

Per Serving:

calorie: 294 | fat: 21g | protein: 14g | carbs: 14g | sugars: 7g | fiber: 4g | sodium: 544mg

Quick Steak Tacos

Prep time: 5 minutes | Cook time: 10 minutes | Serves 6

1 tablespoon olive oil	¾ cup reduced-fat Mexican
8 ounces sirloin steak	cheese
2 tablespoons steak seasoning	2 tablespoons low-fat sour
1 teaspoon Worcestershire sauce	cream
½ red onion, halved and sliced	6 tablespoons garden fresh salsa
6 corn tortillas	¼ cup chopped fresh cilantro
¼ cup tomatoes	

1. Turn the Instant Pot on the Sauté function. When the pot displays "hot," add the olive oil to the pot. 2. Season the steak with the steak seasoning. 3. Add the steak to the pot along with the Worcestershire sauce. 4. Cook each side of the steak for 2–3 minutes until the steak turns brown. 5. Remove the steak from the pot and slice thinly. 6. Add the onion to the pot with the remaining olive oil and steak juices and cook them until translucent. 7. Remove the onion from the pot. 8. Warm your corn tortillas, then assemble your steak, onion, tomatoes, cheese, sour cream, salsa, and cilantro on top of each.

Per Serving:

calories: 187 | fat: 9g | protein: 14g | carbs: 14g | sugars: 2g | fiber: 2g | sodium: 254mg

Spice-Infused Roast Beef

Prep time: 5 minutes | Cook time: 1 hour 30 minutes | Serves 8

¾ cup grated onion, divided	1 tablespoon extra-virgin olive
1 tablespoon caraway seeds	oil
1 teaspoon ground coriander	⅓ cup red wine vinegar
1 teaspoon ground ginger	1 cup unsweetened apple juice
2-pound lean boneless chuck	1 bunch fresh parsley, minced
roast	

1. Preheat the oven to 325 degrees. 2. In a small bowl, combine ¼ cup of the onion, caraway seeds, coriander, and ginger, and rub into the roast. 3. In a medium saucepan over medium heat, sauté the remaining ½ cup of onion in olive oil. Place the roast in a roasting pan, and add the sautéed onion. 4. Add the vinegar, apple juice, parsley, and ½ cup water to the roasting pan. Bake the roast uncovered at 325 degrees for 1–1½ hours, basting frequently. Transfer the roast to a platter, and slice.

Per Serving:

calorie: 194 | fat: 8g | protein: 24g | carbs: 6g | sugars: 4g | fiber: 1g | sodium: 105mg

Mustard Herb Pork Tenderloin

Prep time: 5 minutes | Cook time: 20 minutes | Serves 6

¼ cup mayonnaise	1 (1 pound / 454 g) pork
2 tablespoons Dijon mustard	tenderloin
½ teaspoon dried thyme	½ teaspoon salt
¼ teaspoon dried rosemary	¼ teaspoon ground black pepper

1. In a small bowl, mix mayonnaise, mustard, thyme, and rosemary. Brush tenderloin with mixture on all sides, then sprinkle with salt and pepper on all sides. 2. Place tenderloin into ungreased air fryer basket. Adjust the temperature to 400ºF (204ºC) and air fry for 20 minutes, turning tenderloin halfway through cooking. Tenderloin will be golden and have an internal temperature of at least 145ºF (63ºC) when done. Serve warm.

Per Serving:

calorie: 118 | fat: 5g | protein: 17g | carbs: 1g | sugars: 0g | fiber: 0g | sodium: 368mg

Broiled Dijon Burgers

Prep time: 25 minutes | Cook time: 10 minutes | Makes 6 burgers

¼ cup fat-free egg product or 2	1 cup soft bread crumbs (about
egg whites	2 slices bread)
2 tablespoons fat-free (skim)	1 small onion, finely chopped
milk	(⅓ cup)
2 teaspoons Dijon mustard or	1 pound extra-lean (at least
horseradish sauce	90%) ground beef
¼ teaspoon salt	6 whole-grain burger buns, split,
⅛ teaspoon pepper	toasted

1. Set oven control to broil. Spray broiler pan rack with cooking spray. 2. In medium bowl, mix egg product, milk, mustard, salt and pepper. Stir in bread crumbs and onion. Stir in beef. Shape mixture into 6 patties, each about ½ inch thick. Place patties on rack in broiler pan. 3. Broil with tops of patties about 5 inches from heat 6 minutes. Turn; broil until meat thermometer inserted in center of patties reads 160°F, 4 to 6 minutes longer. Serve patties in buns.

Per Serving:

calories: 250 | fat: 8g | protein: 22g | carbs: 23g | sugars: 5g | fiber: 3g | sodium: 450mg

Pork Tenderloin Stir-Fry

Prep time: 5 minutes | Cook time: 20 minutes | Serves 6

1 tablespoon sesame oil	broth
1-pound pork tenderloin, cut	1 tablespoon light soy sauce
into thin strips	1 cup fresh snow peas, trimmed
1 tablespoon oyster sauce	1 cup broccoli florets
(found in the Asian food section	½ cup sliced water chestnuts,
of the grocery store)	drained
1 tablespoon cornstarch	1 cup diced red pepper
½ cup low-sodium chicken	¼ cup sliced scallions

1. In a large skillet or wok, heat the oil. Stir-fry the pork until the strips are no longer pink. 2. In a measuring cup, combine the oyster sauce, cornstarch, chicken broth, and soy sauce. Add the sauce to the pork, and cook until the sauce thickens. 3. Add the vegetables, cover, and steam for 5 minutes. Serve.

Per Serving:

calorie: 149 | fat: 5g | protein: 18g | carbs: 8g | sugars: 3g | fiber: g | sodium: 174mg

Steak Fajita Bake

Prep time: 10 minutes | Cook time: 15 minutes | Serves 4

1 green bell pepper

1 yellow bell pepper

1 red bell pepper

1 small white onion

10 ounces sirloin steak, trimmed of visible fat

2 tablespoons avocado oil

½ teaspoon ground cumin

¼ teaspoon chili powder

¼ teaspoon garlic powder

4 (6-inch) 100% whole-wheat tortillas

1. Preheat the oven to 400ºF. 2. Cut the green bell pepper, yellow bell pepper, red bell pepper, onion, and steak into ½-inch-thick slices, and put them on a large baking sheet. 3. In a small bowl, combine the oil, cumin, chili powder, and garlic powder, then drizzle the mixture over the meat and vegetables to fully coat them. 4. Arrange the steak and vegetables in a single layer, and bake for 10 to 15 minutes, or until the steak is cooked through. 5. Divide the steak and vegetables equally between the tortillas.

Per Serving:

calorie: 360 | fat: 19g | protein: 20g | carbs: 27g | sugars: 4g | fiber: 6g | sodium: 257mg

Butterflied Beef Eye Roast

Prep time: 10 minutes | Cook time: 40 minutes | Serves 12

3 pounds lean beef eye roast

3 tablespoons extra-virgin olive oil

¼ cup water

½ cup red wine vinegar

3 garlic cloves, minced

½ teaspoon crushed red pepper

1 tablespoon chopped fresh thyme

1. Slice the roast down the middle, open it, and lay it flat in a shallow baking dish. 2. In a small bowl, combine the remaining ingredients, and pour the mixture over the roast. Cover, and let the meat marinate in the refrigerator for at least 12 hours, or up to 24 hours. Turn the roast occasionally. 3. Set the oven to broil. Remove the roast from the marinade, discard the marinade, and place the roast on a rack in the broiler pan. Broil the roast 5 to 7 inches from the heat, turning occasionally, for 20 to 25 minutes or until desired degree of doneness. 4. Remove from the oven, cover with foil, and let stand for 15 to 20 minutes before carving. Transfer to a serving platter, spoon any juices over the top, and serve.

Per Serving:

calorie: 191 | fat: 10g | protein: 24g | carbs: 0g | sugars: 0g | fiber: 0g | sodium: 98mg

Apple Cinnamon Pork Chops

Prep time: 5 minutes | Cook time: 20 minutes | Serves 2

2 teaspoons extra-virgin olive oil

1 large apple, sliced

½ teaspoon organic cinnamon

⅛ teaspoon freshly grated nutmeg

Two 3-ounce lean boneless pork chops, trimmed of fat

1. In a medium nonstick skillet, heat the olive oil. Add the apple slices, and sauté until just tender. Sprinkle with cinnamon and nutmeg, remove from heat, and keep warm. 2. Place the pork chops in the skillet, and cook thoroughly; a meat thermometer inserted into the thickest part of the meat should reach 145 degrees. Remove the pork chops from the skillet, arrange on a serving platter, spoon the apple slices on top, and serve.

Per Serving:

calorie: 208 | fat: 8g | protein: 19g | carbs: 16g | sugars: 11g | fiber: 3g | sodium: 43mg

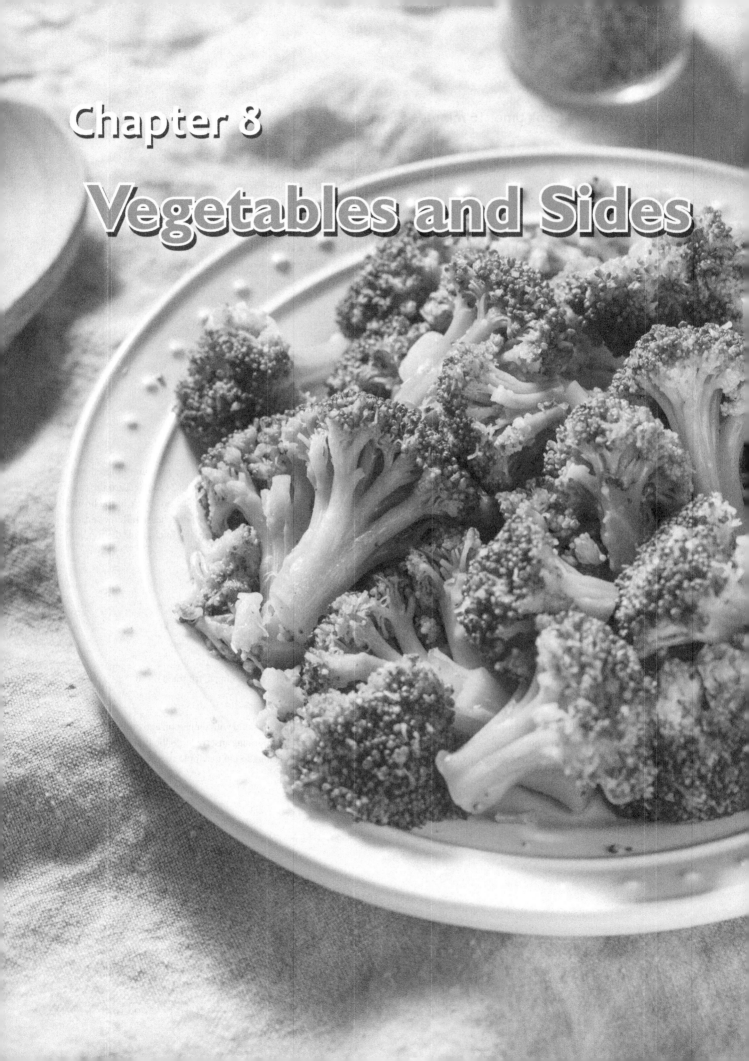

Chapter 8
Vegetables and Sides

Orange-Scented Asparagus with Sweet Red Peppers

Prep time: 5 minutes | Cook time: 15 minutes | Serves 2

⅓ pound fresh asparagus, trimmed	1 tablespoon grated orange zest
1 teaspoon extra-virgin olive oil mixed with 1 teaspoon warm water	Salt, to season
	Freshly ground black pepper, to season
1 red bell pepper, seeded and julienned	1 teaspoon granulated stevia, divided

1. Preheat the broiler to high. 2. In a steamer or large pot of boiling water, cook the asparagus for about 7 minutes, or until barely tender. Drain. Set aside. 3. In a small skillet set over medium-high heat, heat the olive oil and water. 4. Add the bell pepper. Cook for about 5 minutes, stirring frequently, until slightly softened. Remove from the heat. 5. Stir in the orange zest. Season with salt and pepper. 6. Evenly divided the asparagus between 2 gratin dishes. Spoon half of the red bell pepper and sauce over each. Sprinkle each with ½ teaspoon of stevia. Place the dished under the preheated broiler. Broil for 2 to 3 minutes, or until lightly browned. 7. Serve immediately.

Per Serving:

calories: 59 | fat: 2g | protein: 2g | carbs: 9g | sugars: 5g | fiber: 2g | sodium: 585mg

Lemony Brussels Sprouts with Poppy Seeds

Prep time: 10 minutes | Cook time: 2 minutes | Serves 4

1 pound (454 g) Brussels sprouts	1 tablespoon minced garlic
2 tablespoons avocado oil, divided	½ teaspoon kosher salt
	Freshly ground black pepper, to taste
1 cup vegetable broth or chicken bone broth	½ medium lemon
	½ tablespoon poppy seeds

1. Trim the Brussels sprouts by cutting off the stem ends and removing any loose outer leaves. Cut each in half lengthwise (through the stem). 2. Set the electric pressure cooker to the Sauté/More setting. When the pot is hot, pour in 1 tablespoon of the avocado oil. 3. Add half of the Brussels sprouts to the pot, cut-side down, and let them brown for 3 to 5 minutes without disturbing. Transfer to a bowl and add the remaining tablespoon of avocado oil and the remaining Brussels sprouts to the pot. Hit Cancel and return all of the Brussels sprouts to the pot. 4. Add the broth, garlic, salt, and a few grinds of pepper. Stir to distribute the seasonings. 5. Close and lock the lid of the pressure cooker. Set the valve to sealing. 6. Cook on high pressure for 2 minutes. 7. While the Brussels sprouts are cooking, zest the lemon, then cut it into quarters. 8. When the cooking is complete, hit Cancel and quick release the pressure. 9. Once the pin drops, unlock and remove the lid. 10. Using a slotted spoon, transfer the Brussels sprouts to a serving bowl. Toss with the lemon zest, a squeeze of lemon juice, and the poppy seeds. Serve immediately.

Per Serving:

calories: 125 | fat: 8g | protein: 4g | carbs: 13g | sugars: 3g | fiber: 5g | sodium: 504mg

Broccoli with Pine Nuts

Prep time: 10 minutes | Cook time: 5 minutes | Serves 2

1 bunch broccoli rabe	1 tablespoon freshly squeezed lemon juice
4 cups water	
1 cup broccoli florets	Salt, to season
1 tablespoon extra-virgin olive oil	Freshly ground black pepper, to season
2 medium garlic cloves, minced	2 tablespoons pine nuts

1. Rinse the broccoli rabe well in cold water to remove any dirt particles. Tear into stalks. Set aside. 2. In a saucepan set over high heat, bring the water to a boil. 3. Place a colander in the sink. Add the broccoli rabe pieces and broccoli florets. Pour the boiling water over them to scald. Drain well. Set aside. 4. In a sauté pan or skillet set over medium heat, heat the olive oil. 5. Add the garlic. Sauté for 1 minute, or until browned. 6. Add the broccoli rabe and broccoli florets. Toss to coat with the garlic. Cook for about 3 minutes, or until heated through. 7. Drizzle the vegetables with the lemon juice. Season with salt and pepper. 8. Top with the pine nuts and serve.

Per Serving:

calories: 152 | fat: 8g | protein: 10g | carbs: 11g | sugars: 2g | fiber: 7g | sodium: 724mg

Lean Green Avocado Mashed Potatoes

Prep time: 15 minutes | Cook time: 30 minutes | Serves 4

2 large russet potatoes, chopped	rosemary
1 large head cauliflower, cut into 1-inch (2½ cm) florets	1 tablespoon (3 g) dried thyme
	2 cloves garlic
2 medium leeks, washed and coarsely chopped	1 medium avocado, peeled and pitted
2 teaspoons (10 ml) olive oil	2 tablespoons (8 g) finely chopped fresh chives
1 tablespoon (3 g) dried	

1. Preheat the oven to 400°F (204°C). 2. Spread out the potatoes, cauliflower, and leeks on a large baking sheet. Drizzle the vegetables with the oil, then sprinkle them with the rosemary and thyme. Add the garlic to the baking sheet. Bake the vegetables for about 30 minutes, until the potatoes are fork-tender. 3. Transfer the vegetables to a food processor and add the avocado. Process the mixture to the desired consistency. 4. Top the mashed potatoes with the chives and serve.

Per Serving:

calorie: 248 | fat: 10g | protein: 7g | carbs: 37g | sugars: 6g | fiber: 9g | sodium: 69mg

Roasted Eggplant

Prep time: 15 minutes | Cook time: 15 minutes | Serves 4

1 large eggplant	¼ teaspoon salt
2 tablespoons olive oil	½ teaspoon garlic powder

1. Remove top and bottom from eggplant. Slice eggplant into ¼-inch-thick round slices. 2. Brush slices with olive oil. Sprinkle with salt and garlic powder. Place eggplant slices into the air fryer basket. 3. Adjust the temperature to 390ºF (199ºC) and set the timer for 15 minutes. 4. Serve immediately.

Per Serving:

calories: 98 | fat: 7g | protein: 2g | carbs: 8g | sugars: 3g | fiber: 3g | sodium: 200mg

Cauliflower Rice

Prep time: 5 minutes | Cook time: 5 minutes | Makes 2½ cups

1½ pounds cauliflower, coarsely chopped	oil
½ tablespoon extra-virgin olive	Kosher salt
	Freshly ground black pepper

1. Pulse the cauliflower in a food processor until it has a crumbly texture, almost like rice. Be careful not to over-pulse and make it too fine. It's okay to have some larger chunks. Another option is to use a box grater if you don't have a food processor. Put the crumbled cauliflower in a bowl and set aside. 2. Heat the oil in a large skillet over medium-high heat. Add the cauliflower, coat it with hot oil, and sauté 3 to 5 minutes. Season with salt and pepper and serve. 3. Store any leftovers in an airtight container in the refrigerator for 3 to 4 days.

Per Serving:

calories: 118 | fat: 4g | protein: 7g | carbs: 18g | sugars: 7g | fiber: 7g | sodium: 684mg

Mushroom "Bacon" Topper

Prep time: 10 minutes | Cook time: 16 to 17 minutes | Serves 4

½ pound shiitake mushrooms, stems removed	½ teaspoon smoked paprika
2½ teaspoons balsamic vinegar	½ teaspoon Dijon mustard
2½ teaspoons tamari	¼ teaspoon liquid smoke
1 tablespoon pure maple syrup	Freshly ground pepper or lemon pepper to taste

1. Preheat the oven to 400°F. Line a baking sheet with parchment paper. 2. Use a damp paper towel to clean the mushrooms. Slice the mushrooms thinly. In a large bowl, combine the vinegar, tamari, syrup, paprika, mustard, liquid smoke, and pepper. Whisk thoroughly. Add the mushrooms and stir to coat with the marinade. Transfer the mushrooms to the prepared baking sheet. Bake for 16 to 17 minutes, tossing once. Turn off the heat and let the mushrooms sit in the warm oven for 10 minutes, tossing once during this time. Remove and let cool. Serve on salads, soups, pizzas, and more.

Per Serving:

calorie: 45 | fat: 0g | protein: 2g | carbs: 9g | sugars: 6g | fiber: 2g | sodium: 233mg

Green Beans with Red Peppers

Prep time: 5 minutes | Cook time: 15 minutes | Serves 2

8 ounces fresh green beans, broken into 2-inch pieces	into ¼-inch strips
6 sun-dried tomatoes (not packed in oil), halved	1 teaspoon extra-virgin olive oil
1 medium red bell pepper, cut	Salt, to season
	Freshly ground black pepper, to season

1. In a 1-quart saucepan set over high heat, add the green beans to 1 inch of water. Bring to a boil. Boil for 5 minutes, uncovered. 2. Add the sun-dried tomatoes. Cover and boil 5 to 7 minutes more, or until the beans are crisp-tender, and the tomatoes have softened. Drain. Transfer to a serving bowl. 3. Add the red bell pepper and olive oil. Season with salt and pepper. Toss to coat. 4. Serve warm.

Per Serving:

calories: 82 | fat: 3g | protein: 3g | carbs: 13g | sugars: 6g | fiber: 4g | sodium: 601mg

Green Bean and Radish Potato Salad

Prep time: 10 minutes | Cook time: 20 minutes | Serves 6

Kosher salt	lemon juice
6 ounces fresh green beans, trimmed and cut into 1-inch pieces	1 tablespoon Dijon or whole-grain mustard
1½ pounds fingerling potatoes	1 shallot, minced
⅓ cup extra-virgin olive oil	8 radishes, thinly sliced
2 tablespoons freshly squeezed	¼ cup fresh dill, chopped
	Freshly ground black pepper

1. Place a small saucepan filled three-quarters full of water and a pinch of salt over high heat and bring it to a boil. Add the green beans and boil for 2 minutes, then transfer them with a slotted spoon to a colander. Run the beans under cold running water until cool and transfer to a medium bowl. 2. Place the potatoes in the same pot of boiling water, reduce the heat to low, and simmer until tender, about 12 minutes. 3. Meanwhile, combine the extra-virgin olive oil, lemon juice, mustard, and shallot in a jar. Seal with the lid and shake vigorously. If you don't have a jar with a fitted lid, you can also whisk the ingredients in a bowl. 4. Transfer the cooked potatoes to a colander and cool them under cold running water. When they're cool enough to handle, slice the potatoes into thin rounds. 5. Add the potatoes and dressing to the bowl with the green beans, along with the radishes and dill, and toss to combine. 6. Season with salt and pepper and serve. 7. Store any leftovers in an airtight container in the refrigerator for 3 to 4 days.

Per Serving:

calories: 206 | fat: 12g | protein: 3g | carbs: 23g | sugars: 1g | fiber: 3g | sodium: 202mg

Teriyaki Chickpeas

Prep time: 5 minutes | Cook time: 20 to 25 minutes | Serves 7

2 cans (15 ounces each) chickpeas, rinsed and drained	1 tablespoon lemon juice
1½ tablespoons tamari	½ to ¾ teaspoon garlic powder
1 tablespoon pure maple syrup	½ teaspoon ground ginger
	½ teaspoon blackstrap molasses

1. Preheat the oven to 450°F. Line a baking sheet with parchment paper. 2. In a large mixing bowl, combine the chickpeas, tamari, syrup, lemon juice, garlic powder, ginger, and molasses. Toss to combine. Spread evenly on the prepared baking sheet and bake for 20 to 25 minutes, or until the marinade is absorbed. Serve warm, or refrigerate to enjoy later.

Per Serving:

calorie: 120 | fat: 2 | protein: 6g | carbs: 20g | sugars: 5g | fiber: 5g | sodium: 382mg

Cheesy Broiled Tomatoes

Prep time: 5 minutes | Cook time: 10 minutes | Serves 2

2 large ripe tomatoes, halved widthwise	½ teaspoon dried basil, divided
¼ cup nonfat ricotta cheese, divided	Salt, to season
	Freshly ground black pepper, to season

1. Preheat the broiler. 2. Top each tomato half with 1 tablespoon of ricotta cheese. Sprinkle with ⅛ teaspoon of basil. Season with salt and pepper. 3. On a broiler rack, place the tomatoes cut-side up. Place the rack into the preheated oven. Broil for 7 to 10 minutes. 4. Enjoy!

Per Serving:

calories: 49 | fat: 0g | protein: 4g | carbs: 9g | sugars: 5g | fiber: 3g | sodium: 658mg

Blooming Onion

Prep time: 10 minutes | Cook time: 10 minutes | Serves 8

2 Vidalia onions, peeled	1 teaspoon ground cumin
1 cup whole-wheat flour	1 teaspoon Creole seasoning
1 cup chickpea flour	1 cup low-fat buttermilk
2 tablespoons paprika	2 medium egg whites

1. Cut off the top of each onion, then cut each onion vertically until you almost reach the base, taking care not to cut all the way through. Rotate each onion, and make 4 to 6 more vertical cuts to create blooming flowers. 2. In a mixing bowl, use a fork to combine the whole-wheat flour, chickpea flour, paprika, cumin, and Creole seasoning. 3. In another bowl, whisk the buttermilk and egg whites together. 4. Soak the onions in the buttermilk-egg mixture for 60 to 90 seconds, then dredge in the flour mixture. Dunk again in the buttermilk-egg mixture, and place the coated onion in the basket of an air fryer. 5. Set the air fryer to 390°F, close, and cook for 10 minutes. 6. Serve with a plate of greens.

Per Serving:

calories: 135 | fat: 2g | protein: 7g | carbs: 23g | sugars: 4g | fiber: 4g | sodium: 82mg

Bacon-Wrapped Asparagus

Prep time: 10 minutes | Cook time: 10 minutes | Serves 4

8 slices reduced-sodium bacon, cut in half	g) asparagus spears, trimmed of woody ends
16 thick (about 1 pound / 454	

1. Preheat the air fryer to 350°F (177°C). 2. Wrap a half piece of bacon around the center of each stalk of asparagus. 3. Working in batches, if necessary, arrange seam-side down in a single layer in the air fryer basket. Air fry for 10 minutes until the bacon is crisp and the stalks are tender.

Per Serving:

calories: 146 | fat: 10g | protein: 12g | carbs: 4g | sugars: 2g | fiber: 2g | sodium: 502mg

Classic Oven-Roasted Carrots

Prep time: 10 minutes | Cook time: 15 minutes | Serves 4

1½ pounds (680 g) large carrots, trimmed and washed	¼ teaspoon sea salt
Avocado oil spray, as needed	1 tablespoon (3 g) dried rosemary

1. Preheat the oven to 400°F (204°C). Line a large baking sheet with parchment paper. 2. Arrange the carrots on the prepared baking sheet, making sure there is at least ½ inch (13 mm) between each of them. 3. Generously spray the carrots with the avocado oil spray, and then sprinkle them with the sea salt and rosemary. Roast the carrots for 15 minutes, or until they are fork-tender.

Per Serving:

calorie: 72 | fat: 1g | protein: 2g | carbs: 17g | sugars: 8g | fiber: 5g | sodium: 263mg

Sweet-and-Sour Cabbage Slaw

Prep time: 10 minutes | Cook time: 0 minutes | Serves 2

2 tablespoons apple cider vinegar	1 tart apple, cored and diced
1 tablespoon granulated stevia	½ cup shredded carrot
2 cups angel hair cabbage	2 medium scallions, sliced
	2 tablespoons sliced almonds

1. In a medium bowl, stir together the vinegar and stevia. 2. In a large bowl, mix together the cabbage, apple, carrot, and scallions. 3. Pour the sweetened vinegar over the vegetable mixture. Toss to combine. 4. Garnish with the sliced almonds and serve.

Per Serving:

calories: 125 | fat: 1g | protein: 2g | carbs: 30g | sugars: 21g | fiber: 5g | sodium: 47mg

Garlicky Cabbage and Collard Greens

Prep time: 10 minutes | Cook time: 10 minutes | Serves 8

2 tablespoons extra-virgin olive oil

1 collard greens bunch, stemmed and thinly sliced

½ small green cabbage, thinly sliced

6 garlic cloves, minced

1 tablespoon low-sodium gluten-free soy sauce or tamari

1. In a large skillet, heat the oil over medium-high heat. 2. Add the collards to the pan, stirring to coat with oil. Sauté for 1 to 2 minutes until the greens begin to wilt. 3. Add the cabbage and stir to coat. Cover and reduce the heat to medium low. Continue to cook for 5 to 7 minutes, stirring once or twice, until the greens are tender. 4. Add the garlic and soy sauce and stir to incorporate. Cook until just fragrant, about 30 seconds longer. Serve warm and enjoy!

Per Serving:
calories: 72| fat: 4g | protein: 3g | carbs: 6g | sugars: 0g | fiber: 3g | sodium: 129mg

Sautéed Mixed Vegetables

Prep time: 20 minutes | Cook time: 8 minutes | Serves 4

2 teaspoons extra-virgin olive oil

2 carrots, peeled and sliced

4 cups broccoli florets

4 cups cauliflower florets

1 red bell pepper, seeded and cut into long strips

1 cup green beans, trimmed

Sea salt

Freshly ground black pepper

1. Place a large skillet over medium heat and add the olive oil. 2. Sauté the carrots, broccoli, and cauliflower until tender-crisp, about 6 minutes. 3. Add the bell pepper and green beans, and sauté 2 minutes more. 4. Season with salt and pepper, and serve.

Per Serving:
calories: 97 | fat: 3g | protein: 5g | carbs: 15g | sugars: 5g | fiber: 6g | sodium: 211mg

Spicy Roasted Cauliflower with Lime

Prep time: 5 minutes | Cook time: 10 minutes | Serves 4

1 cauliflower head, broken into small florets

2 tablespoons extra-virgin olive oil

½ teaspoon ground chipotle chili powder

½ teaspoon salt

Juice of 1 lime

1. Preheat the oven to 450°F. Line a rimmed baking sheet with parchment paper. 2. In a large mixing bowl, toss the cauliflower with the olive oil, chipotle chili powder, and salt. Arrange in a single layer on the prepared baking sheet. 3. Roast for 15 minutes, flip, and continue to roast for 15 more minutes until well-browned and tender.

4. Sprinkle with the lime juice, adjust the salt as needed, and serve.

Per Serving:
calories: 99 | fat: 7 | protein: 3g | carbs: 8g | sugars: 3g | fiber: 3g | sodium: 284mg

Chipotle Twice-Baked Sweet Potatoes

Prep time: 20 minutes | Cook time: 1 hour | Serves 4

4 small sweet potatoes (about 1¾ pounds)

¼ cup fat-free half-and-half

1 chipotle chile in adobo sauce (from 7 ounces can), finely chopped

1 teaspoon adobo sauce (from

can of chipotle chiles)

½ teaspoon salt

8 teaspoons reduced-fat sour cream

4 teaspoons chopped fresh cilantro

1. Heat oven to 375°F. Gently scrub potatoes but do not peel. Pierce potatoes several times with fork to allow steam to escape while potatoes bake. Bake about 45 minutes or until potatoes are tender when pierced in center with a fork. 2. When potatoes are cool enough to handle, cut lengthwise down through center of potato to within ½ inch of ends and bottom. Carefully scoop out inside, leaving thin shell. In medium bowl, mash potatoes, half-and-half, chile, adobo sauce and salt with potato masher or electric mixer on low speed until light and fluffy. 3. Increase oven temperature to 400°F. In 13x9-inch pan, place potato shells. Divide potato mixture evenly among shells. Bake uncovered 20 minutes or until potato mixture is golden brown and heated through. 4. Just before serving, top each potato with 2 teaspoons sour cream and 1 teaspoon cilantro.

Per Serving:
calorie: 140 | fat: 1g | protein: 3g | carbs: 27g | sugars: 9g | fiber: 4g | sodium: 400mg

Broiled Spinach

Prep time: 5 minutes | Cook time: 4 minutes | Serves 4

8 cups spinach, thoroughly washed and spun dry

1 tablespoon extra-virgin olive oil

¼ teaspoon ground cumin

Sea salt

Freshly ground black pepper

1. Preheat the broiler. Put an oven rack in the upper third of the oven. 2. Set a wire rack on a large baking sheet. 3. In a large bowl, massage the spinach, oil, and cumin together until all the leaves are well coated. 4. Spread half the spinach out on the rack, with as little overlap as possible. Season the greens lightly with salt and pepper. 5. Broil the spinach until the edges are crispy, about 2 minutes. 6. Remove the baking sheet from the oven and transfer the spinach to a large serving bowl. 7. Repeat with the remaining spinach. 8. Serve immediately.

Per Serving:
calories: 44 | fat: 4g | protein: 2g | carbs: 2g | sugars: 0g | fiber: 1g | sodium: 193mg

Asparagus-Pepper Stir-Fry

Prep time: 25 minutes | Cook time: 5 minutes | Serves 4

1 pound fresh asparagus spears	2 cloves garlic, finely chopped
1 teaspoon canola oil	1 tablespoon orange juice
1 medium red, yellow or orange bell pepper, cut into ¾-inch pieces	1 tablespoon reduced-sodium soy sauce
	½ teaspoon ground ginger

1. Break off tough ends of asparagus as far down as stalks snap easily. Cut into 1-inch pieces. 2. In 10-inch nonstick skillet or wok, heat oil over medium heat. Add asparagus, bell pepper and garlic; cook 3 to 4 minutes or until crisp-tender, stirring constantly. 3. In small bowl, mix orange juice, soy sauce and ginger until blended; stir into asparagus mixture. Cook and stir 15 to 30 seconds or until vegetables are coated.

Per Serving:

calorie: 40 | fat: 2g | protein: 2g | carbs: 6g | sugars: 3g | fiber: 2g | sodium: 135mg

Herb-Roasted Root Vegetables

Prep time: 15 minutes | Cook time: 45 to 55 minutes | Serves 6

2 medium turnips, peeled, cut into 1-inch pieces (3 cups)	1 cup ready-to-eat baby-cut carrots
2 medium parsnips, peeled, cut into ½-inch pieces (1½ cups)	Cooking spray
1 medium red onion, cut into 1-inch wedges (1 cup)	2 teaspoons Italian seasoning
	½ teaspoon coarse salt

1 Heat oven to 425°F. Spray 15x10x1-inch pan with cooking spray. Arrange vegetables in single layer in pan. Spray with cooking spray (2 or 3 seconds). Sprinkle with Italian seasoning and salt. 2 Bake uncovered 45 to 55 minutes, stirring once, until vegetables are tender.

Per Serving:

calorie: 70 | fat: 0g | protein: 1g | carbs: 15g | sugars: 7g | fiber: 4g | sodium: 260mg

Chinese Asparagus

Prep time: 5 minutes | Cook time: 5 minutes | Serves 4

1 pound asparagus	2 teaspoons cornstarch
½ cup plus 1 tablespoon water, divided	1 tablespoon canola oil
1 tablespoon light soy sauce	2 teaspoons grated fresh ginger
1 tablespoon rice vinegar	1 scallion, minced

1. Trim the tough ends off the asparagus. Cut the stalks diagonally into 2-inch pieces. 2. In a small bowl, combine the ½ cup water, soy sauce, and rice vinegar. 3. In a measuring cup, combine the cornstarch and 1 tablespoon water. Set aside. 4. Heat the oil in a wok or skillet. Add the ginger and scallions, and stir-fry for 30 seconds.

Add the asparagus and stir-fry for a few seconds more. Add the broth mixture, and bring to a boil. Cover, and simmer for 3–5 minutes, until the asparagus is just tender. 5. Add the cornstarch mixture, and cook until thickened. Serve.

Per Serving:

calories: 73 | fat: 4g | protein: 3g | carbs: 7g | sugars: 3g | fiber: 3g | sodium: 64mg

Sautéed Sweet Peppers

Prep time: 5 minutes | Cook time: 10 minutes | Serves 6

1 tablespoon extra-virgin olive oil	¼ teaspoon salt
2 medium green bell peppers, cut into 1-inch squares	⅛ teaspoon freshly ground black pepper
2 medium red bell peppers, cut into 1-inch squares	2 tablespoons finely chopped fresh basil or oregano
2 tablespoons water	2 cups precooked brown rice, hot

1. In a large skillet over medium heat, heat the oil. Add the peppers, and sauté for 3–5 minutes, stirring frequently. 2. Add the water, salt, and pepper; continue sautéing for 4–5 minutes or until the peppers are just tender. Stir in the basil, and remove from the heat. 3. Spread the rice over a serving platter, spoon the peppers and liquid on top, and serve.

Per Serving:

calories: 111 | fat: 3g | protein: 2g | carbs: 19g | sugars: 3g | fiber: 2g | sodium: 103mg

Zucchini Noodles with Lime-Basil Pesto

Prep time: 20 minutes | Cook time: 0 minutes | Serves 4

2 cups packed fresh basil leaves	pepper
½ cup pine nuts	¼ cup extra-virgin olive oil
2 teaspoons minced garlic	4 green or yellow zucchini,
Zest and juice of 1 lime	rinsed, dried, and julienned or
Pinch sea salt	spiralized
Pinch freshly ground black	1 tomato, diced

1. Place the basil, pine nuts, garlic, lime zest, lime juice, salt, and pepper in a food processor or a blender and pulse until very finely chopped. 2. While the machine is running, add the olive oil in a thin stream until a thick paste forms. 3. In a large bowl, combine the zucchini noodles and tomato. Add the pesto by the tablespoonful until you have the desired flavor. Serve the zucchini pasta immediately. 4. Store any leftover pesto in a sealed container in the refrigerator for up to 2 weeks.

Per Serving:

calories: 247 | fat: 25g | protein: 3g | carbs: 5g | sugars: 2g | fiber: 1g | sodium: 148mg

Fennel and Chickpeas

Prep time: 10 minutes | Cook time: 20 minutes | Serves 6

1 tablespoon extra-virgin olive oil	1 cup low-sodium chicken broth
1 small fennel bulb, trimmed and cut into ¼-inch-thick slices	2 teaspoons chopped fresh thyme
1 sweet onion, thinly sliced	¼ teaspoon sea salt
1 (15½-ounce) can sodium-free chickpeas, rinsed and drained	¼ teaspoon freshly ground black pepper
	1 tablespoon butter

1. Place a large saucepan over medium-high heat and add the oil. 2. Sauté the fennel and onion until tender and lightly browned, about 10 minutes. 3. Add the chickpeas, broth, thyme, salt, and pepper. 4. Cover and cook, stirring occasionally, for 10 minutes, until the liquid has reduced by about half. 5. Remove the pan from the heat and stir in the butter. 6. Serve hot.

Per Serving:

calories: 132 | fat: 6g | protein:5 g | carbs: 17g | sugars: 6g | fiber: 4g | sodium: 239mg

Vegetable Medley

Prep time: 20 minutes | Cook time: 2 minutes | Serves 8

2 medium parsnips	1 teaspoon salt
4 medium carrots	3 tablespoons sugar
1 turnip, about 4½ inches diameter	2 tablespoons canola or olive oil
1 cup water	½ teaspoon salt

1. Clean and peel vegetables. Cut in 1-inch pieces. 2. Place the cup of water and 1 teaspoon salt into the Instant Pot's inner pot with the vegetables. 3. Secure the lid and make sure vent is set to sealing. Press Manual and set for 2 minutes. 4. When cook time is up, release the pressure manually and press Cancel. Drain the water from the inner pot. 5. Press Sauté and stir in sugar, oil, and salt. Cook until sugar is dissolved. Serve.

Per Serving:

calories: 63 | fat: 2g | protein: 1g | carbs: 12g | sugars: 6g | fiber: 2g | sodium: 327mg

Dandelion Greens with Sweet Onion

Prep time: 15 minutes | Cook time: 15 minutes | Serves 4

1 tablespoon extra-virgin olive oil	vegetable broth
1 Vidalia onion, thinly sliced	2 bunches dandelion greens, roughly chopped
2 garlic cloves, minced	Freshly ground black pepper
½ cup store-bought low-sodium	

1. In a large skillet, heat the olive oil over low heat. 2. Add the onion and garlic and cook, stirring to prevent the garlic from scorching, for 2 to 3 minutes, or until the onion is translucent. 3. Add the broth and greens and cook, stirring often, for 5 to 7 minutes, or until the greens are wilted. 4. Season with pepper, and serve warm.

Per Serving:

calories: 53 | fat: 4g | protein: 1g | carbs: 5g | sugars: 1g | fiber: 1g | sodium: 39mg

Parmesan Cauliflower Mash

Prep time: 7 minutes | Cook time: 5 minutes | Serves 4

1 head cauliflower, cored and cut into large florets	¾ cup freshly grated Parmesan cheese
½ teaspoon kosher salt	1 tablespoon unsalted butter or ghee (optional)
½ teaspoon garlic pepper	Chopped fresh chives
2 tablespoons plain Greek yogurt	

1. Pour 1 cup of water into the electric pressure cooker and insert a steamer basket or wire rack. 2. Place the cauliflower in the basket. 3. Close and lock the lid of the pressure cooker. Set the valve to sealing. 4. Cook on high pressure for 5 minutes. 5. When the cooking is complete, hit Cancel and quick release the pressure. 6. Once the pin drops, unlock and remove the lid. 7. Remove the cauliflower from the pot and pour out the water. Return the cauliflower to the pot and add the salt, garlic pepper, yogurt, and cheese. Use an immersion blender or potato masher to purée or mash the cauliflower in the pot. 8. Spoon into a serving bowl, and garnish with butter (if using) and chives.

Per Serving:

calories: 141 | fat: 6g | protein: 12g | carbs: 12g | sugars: 9g | fiber: 4g | sodium: 592mg

Ginger Broccoli

Prep time: 10 minutes | Cook time: 10 minutes | Serves 4

1 tablespoon extra-virgin olive oil	florets
½ sweet onion, thinly sliced	¼ cup low-sodium chicken broth
2 teaspoons grated fresh ginger	Sea salt
1 teaspoon minced fresh garlic	Freshly ground black pepper
2 heads broccoli, cut into small	

1. Place a large skillet over medium-high heat and add the oil. 2. Sauté the onion, ginger, and garlic until softened, about 3 minutes. 3. Add the broccoli florets and chicken broth, and sauté until the broccoli is tender, about 5 minutes. 4. Season with salt and pepper. 5. Serve immediately.

Per Serving:

calories: 240 | fat: 6g | protein: 17g | carbs: 41g | sugars: 12g | fiber: 15g | sodium: 341mg

Garlic Roasted Radishes

Prep time: 5 minutes | Cook time: 15 minutes | Serves 2 to 4

1 pound radishes, halved
1 tablespoon canola oil
Pinch kosher salt

4 garlic cloves, thinly sliced
¼ cup chopped fresh dill

1. Preheat the oven to 425°F. Line a baking sheet with parchment paper. 2. In a medium bowl, toss the radishes with the canola oil and salt. Spread the vegetables on the prepared baking sheet and roast for 10 minutes. Remove the sheet from the oven, add the garlic, mix well, and return to the oven for 5 minutes. 3. Remove the radishes from the oven, adjust the seasoning as desired, and serve topped with dill on a serving plate or as a side dish. 4. Store any leftovers in an airtight container in the refrigerator for 3 to 4 days.

Per Serving:

calories: 75 | fat: 5g | protein: 1g | carbs: 8g | sugars: 4g | fiber: 3g | sodium: 420mg

Carrots Marsala

Prep time: 5 minutes | Cook time: 10 minutes | Serves 6

10 carrots (about 1 pound), peeled and diagonally sliced
¼ cup Marsala wine
¼ cup water

1 tablespoon extra-virgin olive oil
⅛ teaspoon freshly ground black pepper
1 tablespoon finely chopped fresh parsley

1. In a large saucepan, combine the carrots, wine, water, oil, and pepper. Bring to a boil, cover, reduce the heat, and simmer for 8 to 10 minutes, until the carrots are just tender, basting occasionally. Taste, and add salt, if desired. 2. Transfer to a serving dish, spoon any juices on top, and sprinkle with parsley.

Per Serving:

calories: 48 | fat: 2g | protein: 1g | carbs: 6g | sugars: 3g | fiber: 2g | sodium: 46mg

Garlic Herb Radishes

Prep time: 10 minutes | Cook time: 10 minutes | Serves 4

1 pound (454 g) radishes
2 tablespoons unsalted butter, melted
½ teaspoon garlic powder

½ teaspoon dried parsley
¼ teaspoon dried oregano
¼ teaspoon ground black pepper

1. Remove roots from radishes and cut into quarters. 2. In a small bowl, add butter and seasonings. Toss the radishes in the herb butter and place into the air fryer basket. 3. Adjust the temperature to 350ºF (177ºC) and set the timer for 10 minutes. 4. Halfway through the cooking time, toss the radishes in the air fryer basket. Continue cooking until edges begin to turn brown. 5. Serve warm.

Per Serving:

calories: 57 | fat: 4g | protein: 1g | carbs: 5g | sugars: 3g | fiber: 2g | sodium: 27mg

Zucchini Ribbons with Tarragon

Prep time: 5 minutes | Cook time: 1 minutes | Serves 2

1 zucchini, thinly sliced lengthwise into ribbons
1 tablespoon nonfat ricotta cheese
1 tablespoon pine nuts

1 tablespoon fresh tarragon
1½ teaspoons extra-virgin olive oil
½ to 1 teaspoon red pepper flakes

1. Bring a large pot of water to a boil. 2. Add the zucchini. Cook for 30 to 60 seconds, or until crisp-tender. Drain. Transfer the zucchini to a serving bowl. 3. Add the ricotta cheese, pine nuts, tarragon, olive oil, and red pepper flakes. Gently toss until the zucchini is coated. 4. Serve and enjoy!

Per Serving:

calories: 62 | fat: 5g | protein: 2g | carbs: 3g | sugars: 1g | fiber: 1g | sodium: 15mg

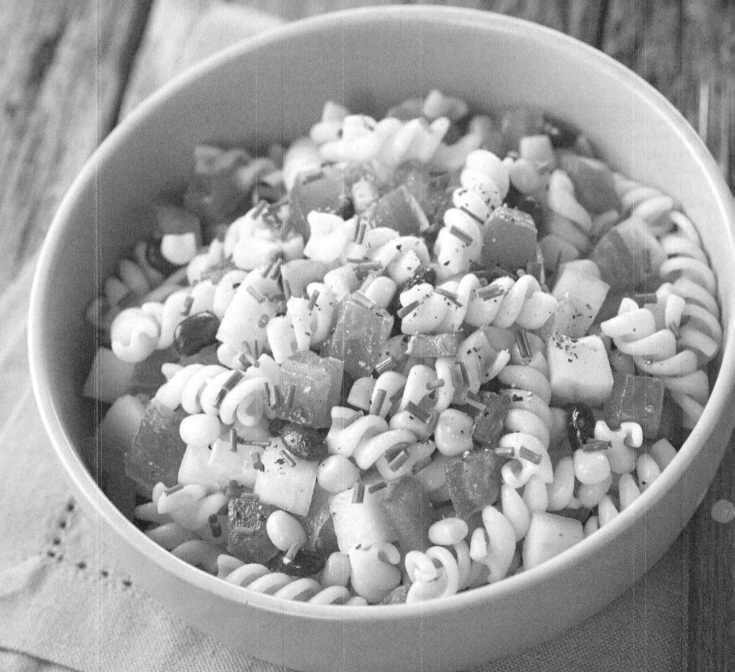

Chapter 9
Vegetarian Mains

Chickpea-Spinach Curry

Prep time: 5 minutes | Cook time: 10 minutes | Serves 2

1 cup frozen chopped spinach, thawed	chopped tomatoes, undrained
1 cup canned chickpeas, drained and rinsed	1 tablespoon curry powder
½ cup frozen green beans	1 tablespoon granulated garlic
½ cup frozen broccoli florets	Salt, to season
½ cup no-salt-added canned	Freshly ground black pepper, to season
	½ cup chopped fresh parsley

1. In a medium saucepan set over high heat, stir together the spinach, chickpeas, green beans, broccoli, tomatoes and their juice, curry powder, and garlic. Season with salt and pepper. Bring to a fast boil. Reduce the heat to low. Cover and simmer for 10 minutes, or until heated through. 2. Top with the parsley, serve, and enjoy!

Per Serving:

calories: 203 | fat: 3g | protein: 13g | carbs: 35g | sugars: 7g | fiber: 13g | sodium: 375mg

Roasted Veggie Bowl

Prep time: 10 minutes | Cook time: 15 minutes | Serves 2

1 cup broccoli florets	seeded and sliced ¼ inch thick
1 cup quartered Brussels sprouts	1 tablespoon coconut oil
½ cup cauliflower florets	2 teaspoons chili powder
¼ medium white onion, peeled and sliced ¼ inch thick	½ teaspoon garlic powder
½ medium green bell pepper,	½ teaspoon cumin

1. Toss all ingredients together in a large bowl until vegetables are fully coated with oil and seasoning. 2. Pour vegetables into the air fryer basket. 3. Adjust the temperature to 360°F (182°C) and roast for 15 minutes. 4. Shake two or three times during cooking. Serve warm.

Per Serving:

calories: 112 | fat: 8g | protein: 4g | carbs: 11g | sugars: 3g | fiber: 5g | sodium: 106mg

No-Tuna Lettuce Wraps

Prep time: 10 minutes | Cook time: 0 minutes | Serves 4

1 (15-ounce) can low-sodium chickpeas, drained and rinsed	red onion
1 celery stalk, thinly sliced	2 tablespoons unsalted tahini
3 tablespoons honey mustard	1 tablespoon capers, undrained
2 tablespoons finely chopped	12 butter lettuce leaves

1. In a large bowl, mash the chickpeas. 2. Add the celery, honey mustard, onion, tahini, and capers, and mix well. 3. For each serving, place three lettuce leaves on a plate so they overlap, top with one-fourth of the chickpea filling, and roll up into a wrap. Repeat with the remaining lettuce leaves and filling.

Per Serving:

calories: 163 | fat: 8g | protein: 6g | carbs: 17g | sugars: 4g | fiber: 6g | sodium: 333mg

Cashew-Kale and Chickpeas

Prep time: 15 minutes | Cook time: 15 minutes | Serves 2

For the cashew sauce	and rinsed
½ cup unsalted cashews soaked in ½ cup hot water for at least 20 minutes	1 bunch kale, thoroughly washed, central stems removed, leaves thinly sliced (about 2½ cups)
1 cup reduced-sodium vegetable broth	2 to 3 tablespoons water
1 garlic clove, minced	1 teaspoon red pepper flakes
For the kale	½ teaspoon salt
1 medium red bell pepper, diced	Freshly ground black pepper, to season
1 medium carrot, julienned	
½ cup sliced fresh mushrooms	¼ cup minced fresh cilantro
1 cup canned chickpeas, drained	

To make the cashew sauce 1. Drain the cashews. 2. In a blender or food processor, blend together the cashews, vegetable broth, and garlic until completely smooth. Set aside. To make the kale 1. In a large nonstick skillet or Dutch oven set over medium-low heat, stir together the red bell pepper, carrot, and mushrooms. Cook for 5 to 7 minutes, or until softened. 2. Stir in the chickpeas. Increase the heat to high. 3. Add the kale and the water. Stir to combine. Cover and cook for 5 minutes, or until the kale is tender. 4. Stir in the cashew sauce, red pepper flakes, and salt. Season with pepper. Cook for 2 to 3 minutes more, uncovered, or until the sauce thickens. 5. Garnish with the cilantro before serving. 6. Enjoy!

Per Serving:

calories: 480 | fat: 20g | protein: 20g | carbs: 62g | sugars: 17g | fiber: 15g | sodium: 843mg

Chickpea Coconut Curry

Prep time: 5 minutes | Cook time: 15 minutes | Serves 4

3 cups fresh or frozen cauliflower florets	chickpeas, drained and rinsed
2 cups unsweetened almond milk	1 tablespoon curry powder
1 (15 ounces) can coconut milk	¼ teaspoon ground ginger
1 (15 ounces) can low-sodium	¼ teaspoon garlic powder
	⅛ teaspoon onion powder
	¼ teaspoon salt

1. In a large stockpot, combine the cauliflower, almond milk, coconut milk, chickpeas, curry, ginger, garlic powder, and onion powder. Stir and cover. 2. Cook over medium-high heat for 10 minutes. 3. Reduce the heat to low, stir, and cook for 5 minutes more, uncovered. Season with up to ¼ teaspoon salt.

Per Serving:

calories: 225 | fat: 7g | protein: 12g | carbs: 31g | sugars: 14g | fiber: 9g | sodium: 489mg

Spinach Salad with Eggs, Tempeh Bacon, and Strawberries

Prep time: 10 minutes | Cook time: 15 minutes | Serves 4

2 tablespoons soy sauce, tamari, or coconut aminos	3 tablespoons extra-virgin olive oil
1 tablespoon raw apple cider vinegar	1 shallot, minced
1 tablespoon pure maple syrup	1 tablespoon red wine vinegar
½ teaspoon smoked paprika	1 tablespoon balsamic vinegar
Freshly ground black pepper	1 teaspoon Dijon mustard
One 8-ounce package tempeh, cut crosswise into ⅛-inch-thick slices	¼ teaspoon fine sea salt
	One 6-ounce bag baby spinach
	2 hearts romaine lettuce, torn into bite-size pieces
8 large eggs	12 fresh strawberries, sliced

1. In a 1-quart ziplock plastic bag, combine the soy sauce, cider vinegar, maple syrup, paprika, and ½ teaspoon pepper and carefully agitate the bag to mix the ingredients to make a marinade. Add the tempeh, seal the bag, and turn the bag back and forth several times to coat the tempeh evenly with the marinade. Marinate in the refrigerator for at least 2 hours or up to 24 hours. 2. Pour 1 cup water into the Instant Pot and place the wire metal steam rack, an egg rack, or a steamer basket into the pot. Gently place the eggs on top of the rack or in the basket, taking care not to crack them. 3. Secure the lid and set the Pressure Release to Sealing. Select the Steam setting and set the cooking time for 3 minutes at high pressure. (The pot will take about 5 minutes to come up to pressure before the cooking program begins.) 4. While the eggs are cooking, prepare an ice bath. 5. When the cooking program ends, perform a quick pressure release by moving the Pressure Release to Venting. Open the pot and, using tongs, transfer the eggs to the ice bath to cool. 6. Remove the tempeh from the marinade and blot dry between layers of paper towels. Discard the marinade. In a large nonstick skillet over medium-high heat, warm 1 tablespoon of the oil for 2 minutes. Add the tempeh in a single layer and fry, turning once, for 2 to 3 minutes per side, until well browned. Transfer the tempeh to a plate and set aside. 7. Wipe out the skillet and set it over medium heat. Add the remaining 2 tablespoons oil and the shallot and sauté for about 2 minutes, until the shallot is golden brown. Turn off the heat and stir in the red wine vinegar, balsamic vinegar, mustard, salt, and ¼ teaspoon pepper to make a vinaigrette. 8. In a large bowl, combine the spinach and romaine. Pour in the vinaigrette and toss until all of the leaves are lightly coated. Divide the dressed greens evenly among four large serving plates or shallow bowls and arrange the strawberries and fried tempeh on top. Peel the eggs, cut them in half lengthwise, and place them on top of the salads. Top with a couple grinds of pepper and serve right away.

Per Serving:

calorie: 435 | fat: 25g | protein: 29g | carbs: 25g | sugars: 10g | fiber: 5g | sodium: 332mg

Instant Pot Hoppin' John with Skillet Cauli "Rice"

Prep time: 0 minutes | Cook time: 30 minutes | Serves 6

Hoppin' John	diced
1 pound dried black-eyed peas (about 2¼ cups)	½ teaspoon smoked paprika
8⅔ cups water	½ teaspoon dried thyme
1½ teaspoons fine sea salt	½ teaspoon dried sage
2 tablespoons extra-virgin olive oil	¼ teaspoon cayenne pepper
	2 cups low-sodium vegetable broth
2 garlic cloves, minced	Cauli "Rice"
8 ounces shiitake mushrooms, stemmed and chopped, or cremini mushrooms, chopped	1 tablespoon vegan buttery spread or unsalted butter
1 small yellow onion, diced	1 pound riced cauliflower
1 green bell pepper, seeded and diced	½ teaspoon fine sea salt
2 celery stalks, diced	2 green onions, white and green parts, sliced
2 jalapeño chiles, seeded and	Hot sauce (such as Tabasco or Crystal) for serving

1. To make the Hoppin' John: In a large bowl, combine the black-eyed peas, 8 cups of the water, and 1 teaspoon of the salt and stir to dissolve the salt. Let soak for at least 8 hours or up to overnight. 2. Select the Sauté setting on the Instant Pot and heat the oil and garlic for 3 minutes, until the garlic is bubbling but not browned. Add the mushrooms and the remaining ½ teaspoon salt and sauté for 5 minutes, until the mushrooms have wilted and begun to give up their liquid. Add the onion, bell pepper, celery, and jalapeños and sauté for 4 minutes, until the onion is softened. Add the paprika, thyme, sage, and cayenne and sauté for 1 minute. 3. Drain the black-eyed peas and add them to the pot along with the broth and remaining ⅔ cup water. The liquid should just barely cover the beans. (Add an additional splash of water if needed.) 4. Secure the lid and set the Pressure Release to Sealing. Press the Cancel button to reset the cooking program, then select the Bean/Chili, Pressure Cook, or Manual setting and set the cooking time for 5 minutes at high pressure. (The pot will take about 10 minutes to come up to pressure before the cooking program begins.) 5. When the cooking program ends, let the pressure release naturally for 10 minutes, then move the Pressure Release to Venting to release any remaining steam. 6. To make the cauli "rice": While the pressure is releasing, in a large skillet over medium heat, melt the buttery spread. Add the cauliflower and salt and sauté for 3 to 5 minutes, until cooked through and piping hot. (If using frozen riced cauliflower, this may take another 2 minutes or so.) 7. Spoon the cauli "rice" onto individual plates. Open the pot and spoon the black-eyed peas on top of the cauli "rice". Sprinkle with the green onions and serve right away, with the hot sauce on the side.

Per Serving:

calories: 287 | fat: 7g | protein: 23g | carbs: 56g | sugars: 8g | fiber: 24g | sodium: 894mg

Vegetable Burgers

Prep time: 10 minutes | Cook time: 12 minutes | Serves 4

8 ounces (227 g) cremini mushrooms	yellow onion
2 large egg yolks	1 clove garlic, peeled and finely minced
½ medium zucchini, trimmed and chopped	½ teaspoon salt
¼ cup peeled and chopped	¼ teaspoon ground black pepper

1. Place all ingredients into a food processor and pulse twenty times until finely chopped and combined. 2. Separate mixture into four equal sections and press each into a burger shape. Place burgers into ungreased air fryer basket. Adjust the temperature to 375ºF (191ºC) and air fry for 12 minutes, turning burgers halfway through cooking. Burgers will be browned and firm when done. 3. Place burgers on a large plate and let cool 5 minutes before serving.

Per Serving:

calories: 77 | fat: 5g | protein: 3g | carbs: 6g | sugars: 2g | fiber: 1g | sodium: 309mg

Vegan Dal Makhani

Prep time: 0 minutes | Cook time: 55 minutes | Serves 6

1 cup dried kidney beans	diced
⅓ cup urad dal or beluga or Puy lentils	1 tablespoon garam masala
4 cups water	1 teaspoon ground turmeric
1 teaspoon fine sea salt	¼ teaspoon cayenne pepper (optional)
1 tablespoon cold-pressed avocado oil	One 15-ounce can fire-roasted diced tomatoes and liquid
1 tablespoon cumin seeds	2 tablespoons vegan buttery spread
1-inch piece fresh ginger, peeled and minced	Cooked cauliflower "rice" for serving
4 garlic cloves, minced	2 tablespoons chopped fresh cilantro
1 large yellow onion, diced	
2 jalapeño chiles, seeded and diced	6 tablespoons plain coconut yogurt
1 green bell pepper, seeded and	

1. In a medium bowl, combine the kidney beans, urad dal, water, and salt and stir to dissolve the salt. Let soak for 12 hours. 2. Select the Sauté setting on the Instant Pot and heat the oil and cumin seeds for 3 minutes, until the seeds are bubbling, lightly toasted, and aromatic. Add the ginger and garlic and sauté for 1 minute, until bubbling and fragrant. Add the onion, jalapeños, and bell pepper and sauté for 5 minutes, until the onion begins to soften. 3. Add the garam masala, turmeric, cayenne (if using), and the soaked beans and their liquid and stir to mix. Pour the tomatoes and their liquid on top. Do not stir them in. 4. Secure the lid and set the Pressure Release to Sealing. Press the Cancel button to reset the cooking program, then select the Pressure Cook or Manual setting and set the cooking time for 30 minutes at high pressure. (The pot will take about 15 minutes to come up to pressure before the cooking program begins.) 5. When the cooking program ends, let the pressure release naturally for 30 minutes, then move the Pressure Release to Venting to release any remaining steam. Open the pot and stir to combine, then stir in the buttery spread. If you prefer a smoother texture, ladle 1½ cups of the dal into a blender and blend until smooth, about 30 seconds, then stir the blended mixture into the rest of the dal in the pot. 6. Spoon the cauliflower "rice" into bowls and ladle the dal on top. Sprinkle with the cilantro, top with a dollop of coconut yogurt, and serve.

Per Serving:

calorie: 245 | fat: 7g | protein: 11g | carbs: 37g | sugars: 4g | fiber: 10g | sodium: 518mg

Stuffed Portobello Mushrooms

Prep time: 5 minutes | Cook time: 20 minutes | Serves 4

8 large portobello mushrooms	4 cups fresh spinach
3 teaspoons extra-virgin olive oil, divided	1 medium red bell pepper, diced
	¼ cup crumbled feta

1. Preheat the oven to 450ºF. 2. Remove the stems from the mushrooms, and gently scoop out the gills and discard. Coat the mushrooms with 2 teaspoons of olive oil. 3. On a baking sheet, place the mushrooms cap-side down, and roast for 20 minutes. 4. Meanwhile, heat the remaining 1 teaspoon of olive oil in a medium skillet over medium heat. When hot, sauté the spinach and red bell pepper for 8 to 10 minutes, stirring occasionally. 5. Remove the mushrooms from the oven. Drain, if necessary. Spoon the spinach and pepper mix into the mushrooms, and top with feta.

Per Serving:

calories: 91 | fat: 4g | protein: 6g | carbs: 10g | sugars: g | fiber: 4g | sodium: 155mg

Farro Bowl

Prep time: 5 minutes | Cook time: 25 minutes | Serves 4

3 cups water	pepper
1 cup uncooked farro	4 hardboiled eggs, sliced
1 tablespoon extra-virgin olive oil	1 avocado, sliced
1 teaspoon ground cumin	⅓ cup plain low-fat Greek yogurt
½ teaspoon salt	4 lemon wedges
½ teaspoon freshly ground black	

1. In a medium saucepan, bring the water to a boil over high heat. 2. Pour the farro into the boiling water, and stir to submerge the grains. Reduce the heat to medium and cook for 20 minutes. Drain and set aside. 3. Heat a medium skillet over medium-low heat. When hot, pour in the oil, then add the cooked farro, cumin, salt, and pepper. Cook for 3 to 5 minutes, stirring occasionally. 4. Divide the farro into four equal portions, and top each with one-quarter of the eggs, avocado, and yogurt. Add a squeeze of lemon over the top of each portion.

Per Serving:

calories: 330 | fat: 15g | protein: 14g | carbs: 40g | sugars: 6g | fiber: 8g | sodium: 409mg

Crispy Eggplant Rounds

Prep time: 15 minutes | Cook time: 10 minutes | Serves 4

1 large eggplant, ends trimmed, cut into ½-inch slices	cheese crisps, finely ground
½ teaspoon salt	½ teaspoon paprika
2 ounces (57 g) Parmesan 100%	¼ teaspoon garlic powder
	1 large egg

1. Sprinkle eggplant rounds with salt. Place rounds on a kitchen towel for 30 minutes to draw out excess water. Pat rounds dry. 2. In a medium bowl, mix cheese crisps, paprika, and garlic powder. In a separate medium bowl, whisk egg. Dip each eggplant round in egg, then gently press into cheese crisps to coat both sides. 3. Place eggplant rounds into ungreased air fryer basket. Adjust the temperature to 400ºF (204ºC) and air fry for 10 minutes, turning rounds halfway through cooking. Eggplant will be golden and crispy when done. Serve warm.

Per Serving:

calorie: 109 | fat: 6g | protein: 8g | carbs: 7g | sugars: 3g | fiber: 4g | sodium: 545mg

Black-Eyed Pea Sauté with Garlic and Olives

Prep time: 5 minutes | Cook time: 5 minutes | Serves 2

2 teaspoons extra-virgin olive oil	¼ cup water
1 garlic clove, minced	¼ teaspoon salt
½ red onion, chopped	¼ teaspoon freshly ground black pepper
1 cup cooked black-eyed peas; if canned, drain and rinse	6 Kalamata olives, pitted and halved
½ teaspoon dried thyme	

1. In a medium saucepan set over medium heat, stir together the olive oil, garlic, and red onion. Cook for 2 minutes, continuing to stir. 2. Add the black-eyed peas and thyme. Cook for 1 minute. 3. Stir in the water, salt, pepper, and olives. Cook for 2 minutes more, or until heated through.

Per Serving:

calories: 140 | fat: 6g | protein: 5g | carbs: 18g | sugars: 8g | fiber: 5g | sodium: 426mg

Greek Stuffed Eggplant

Prep time: 15 minutes | Cook time: 20 minutes | Serves 2

1 large eggplant	1 cup fresh spinach
2 tablespoons unsalted butter	2 tablespoons diced red bell pepper
¼ medium yellow onion, diced	½ cup crumbled feta
¼ cup chopped artichoke hearts	

1. Slice eggplant in half lengthwise and scoop out flesh, leaving enough inside for shell to remain intact. Take eggplant that was scooped out, chop it, and set aside. 2. In a medium skillet over medium heat, add butter and onion. Sauté until onions begin to soften, about 3 to 5 minutes. Add chopped eggplant, artichokes, spinach, and bell pepper. Continue cooking 5 minutes until peppers soften and spinach wilts. Remove from the heat and gently fold in the feta. 3. Place filling into each eggplant shell and place into the air fryer basket. 4. Adjust the temperature to 320ºF (160ºC) and air fry for 20 minutes. 5. Eggplant will be tender when done. Serve warm.

Per Serving:

calories: 259 | fat: 16g | protein: 10g | carbs: 22g | sugars: 12g | fiber: 10g | sodium: 386mg

Palak Tofu

Prep time: 5 minutes | Cook time: 40 minutes | Serves 4

One 14-ounce package extra-firm tofu, drained	¼ teaspoon cayenne pepper
5 tablespoons cold-pressed avocado oil	One 16-ounce bag frozen chopped spinach
1 yellow onion, diced	⅓ cup water
1-inch piece fresh ginger, peeled and minced	One 14½-ounce can fire-roasted diced tomatoes and their liquid
3 garlic cloves, minced	¼ cup coconut milk
1 teaspoon fine sea salt	2 teaspoons garam masala
½ teaspoon freshly ground black pepper	Cooked brown rice or cauliflower "rice" or whole-grain flatbread for serving

1. Cut the tofu crosswise into eight ½-inch-thick slices. Sandwich the slices between double layers of paper towels or a folded kitchen towel and press firmly to wick away as much moisture as possible. Cut the slices into ½-inch cubes. 2. Select the Sauté setting on the Instant Pot and and heat 4 tablespoons of the oil for 2 minutes. Add the onion and sauté for about 10 minutes, until it begins to brown. 3. While the onion is cooking in the Instant Pot, in a large nonstick skillet over medium-high heat, warm the remaining 1 tablespoon oil. Add the tofu in a single layer and cook without stirring for about 3 minutes, until lightly browned. 4. Using a spatula, turn the cubes over and cook for about 3 minutes more, until browned on the other side. Remove from the heat and set aside. 5. Add the ginger and garlic to the onion in the Instant Pot and sauté for about 2 minutes, until the garlic is bubbling but not browned. Add the sautéed tofu, salt, black pepper, and cayenne and stir gently to combine, taking care not to break up the tofu. Add the spinach and stir gently. Pour in the water and then pour the tomatoes and their liquid over the top in an even layer. Do not stir them in. 6. Secure the lid and set the Pressure Release to Sealing. Press the Cancel button to reset the cooking program, then select the Manual or Pressure Cook setting and set the cooking time for 10 minutes at low pressure. (The pot will take about 15 minutes to come up to pressure before the cooking program begins.) 7. When the cooking program ends, let the pressure release naturally for 10 minutes, then move the Pressure Release to Venting to release any remaining steam. Open the pot, add the coconut milk and garam masala, and stir to combine. 8. Ladle the tofu onto plates or into bowls. Serve piping hot, with the "rice" alongside.

Per Serving:

calories: 345 | fat: 24g | protein: 14g | carbs: 18g | sugars: 5g | fiber: 6g | sodium: 777mg

The Ultimate Veggie Burger

Prep time: 5 minutes | Cook time: 10 minutes | Serves 2

¾ cup shelled edamame	¼ teaspoon ground cumin
¾ cup frozen mixed vegetables, thawed	1 scallion, sliced
3 tablespoons hemp hearts	2 teaspoons chopped fresh cilantro
2 tablespoons quick-cook oatmeal	2 tablespoons coconut flour
¼ teaspoon salt	2 large egg whites
¼ teaspoon onion powder	Extra-virgin olive oil cooking spray

1. In a food processor, combine the edamame, mixed vegetables, hemp hearts, oatmeal, salt, onion powder, cumin, scallion, cilantro, coconut flour, and egg whites. Pulse until blended, but not completely puréed. You want some texture. 2. Spray a nonstick skillet with cooking spray. Place it over medium-high heat. 3. Spoon half of the mixture into the pan. Using the back of a spoon, spread it out to form a patty. Repeat with the remaining half of the mixture. 4. Cook for 3 to 5 minutes, or until golden, and flip. Cook for about 3 minutes more, or until golden. Turn off the heat. 5. Transfer to serving plates and enjoy!

Per Serving:

calories: 154 | fat: 4g | protein: 13g | carbs: 19g | sugars: 4g | fiber: 7g | sodium: 467mg

Easy Cheesy Vegetable Frittata

Prep time: 10 minutes | Cook time: 15 minutes | Serves 2

Extra-virgin olive oil cooking spray	basil
½ cup sliced onion	Pinch freshly ground black pepper
½ cup sliced green bell pepper	½ cup liquid egg substitute
½ cup sliced eggplant	½ cup nonfat cottage cheese
½ cup frozen spinach	¼ cup fat-free evaporated milk
½ cup sliced fresh mushrooms	¼ cup nonfat shredded Cheddar cheese
1 tablespoon chopped fresh	

1. Coat an ovenproof 10-inch skillet with cooking spray. Place it over medium-low heat until hot. 2. Add the onion, green bell pepper, eggplant, spinach, and mushrooms. Sauté for 2 to 3 minutes, or until lightly browned. 3. Add the basil. Season with pepper. Stir to combine. Cook for 2 to 3 minutes more, or until the flavors blend. Remove from the heat. 4. Preheat the broiler. 5. In a blender, combine the egg substitute, cottage cheese, Cheddar cheese, and evaporated milk. Process until smooth. Pour the egg mixture over the vegetables in the skillet. 6. Return the skillet to medium-low heat. Cover and cook for about 5 minutes, or until the bottom sets and the top is still slightly wet. 7. Transfer the ovenproof skillet to the broiler. Broil for 2 to 3 minutes, or until the top is set. 8. Serve one-half of the frittata per person and enjoy!

Per Serving:

calories: 177 | fat: 7g | protein: 17g | carbs: 12g | sugars: 6g | fiber: 3g | sodium: 408mg

Gingered Tofu and Greens

Prep time: 15 minutes | Cook time: 20 minutes | Serves 2

For the marinade	oil, divided
2 tablespoons low-sodium soy sauce	1 tablespoon grated fresh ginger
¼ cup rice vinegar	2 cups coarsely shredded bok choy
⅓ cup water	2 cups coarsely shredded kale, thoroughly washed
1 tablespoon grated fresh ginger	½ cup fresh, or frozen, chopped green beans
1 tablespoon coconut flour	1 tablespoon freshly squeezed lime juice
1 teaspoon granulated stevia	
1 garlic clove, minced	1 tablespoon chopped fresh cilantro
For the tofu and greens	
8 ounces extra-firm tofu, drained, cut into 1-inch cubes	2 tablespoons hemp hearts
3 teaspoons extra-virgin olive	

To make the marinade 1. In a small bowl, whisk together the soy sauce, rice vinegar, water, ginger, coconut flour, stevia, and garlic until well combined. 2. Place a small saucepan set over high heat. Add the marinade. Bring to a boil. Cook for 1 minute. Remove from the heat. To make the tofu and greens 1. In a medium ovenproof pan, place the tofu in a single layer. Pour the marinade over. Drizzle with 1½ teaspoons of olive oil. Let sit for 5 minutes. 2. Preheat the broiler to high. 3. Place the pan under the broiler. Broil the tofu for 7 to 8 minutes, or until lightly browned. Using a spatula, turn the tofu over. Continue to broil for 7 to 8 minutes more, or until browned on this side. 4. In a large wok or skillet set over high heat, heat the remaining 1½ teaspoons of olive oil. 5. Stir in the ginger. 6. Add the bok choy, kale, and green beans. Cook for 2 to 3 minutes, stirring constantly, until the greens wilt. 7. Add the lime juice and cilantro. Remove from the heat. 8. Add the browned tofu with any remaining marinade in the pan to the bok choy, kale, and green beans. Toss gently to combine. 9. Top with the hemp hearts and serve immediately.

Per Serving:

calories: 252 | fat: 14g | protein: 15g | carbs: 20g | sugars: 4g | fiber: 3g | sodium: 679mg

Parmesan Artichokes

Prep time: 10 minutes | Cook time: 10 minutes | Serves 4

2 medium artichokes, trimmed and quartered, center removed	Parmesan cheese
2 tablespoons coconut oil	¼ cup blanched finely ground almond flour
1 large egg, beaten	½ teaspoon crushed red pepper flakes
½ cup grated vegetarian	

1. In a large bowl, toss artichokes in coconut oil and then dip each piece into the egg. 2. Mix the Parmesan and almond flour in a large bowl. Add artichoke pieces and toss to cover as completely as possible, sprinkle with pepper flakes. Place into the air fryer basket. 3. Adjust the temperature to 400ºF (204ºC) and air fry for 10 minutes. 4. Toss the basket two times during cooking. Serve warm.

Per Serving:

calories: 207 | fat: 13g | protein: 10g | carbs: 15g | sugars: 2g | fiber: 5g | sodium: 211mg

Stuffed Portobellos

Prep time: 10 minutes | Cook time: 8 minutes | Serves 4

3 ounces (85 g) cream cheese, softened	leaves
½ medium zucchini, trimmed and chopped	4 large portobello mushrooms, stems removed
¼ cup seeded and chopped red bell pepper	2 tablespoons coconut oil, melted
1½ cups chopped fresh spinach	½ teaspoon salt

1. In a medium bowl, mix cream cheese, zucchini, pepper, and spinach. 2. Drizzle mushrooms with coconut oil and sprinkle with salt. Scoop ¼ zucchini mixture into each mushroom. 3. Place mushrooms into ungreased air fryer basket. Adjust the temperature to 400ºF (204ºC) and air fry for 8 minutes. Portobellos will be tender and tops will be browned when done. Serve warm.

Per Serving:

calories: 154 | fat: 13g | protein: 4g | carbs: 6g | sugars: 3g | fiber: 2g | sodium: 355mg

Chile Relleno Casserole with Salsa Salad

Prep time: 10 minutes | Cook time: 55 minutes | Serves 4

Casserole	2 Roma tomatoes, seeded and diced
½ cup gluten-free flour (such as King Arthur)	1 green bell pepper, seeded and diced
1 teaspoon baking powder	
6 large eggs	½ small yellow onion, diced
½ cup nondairy milk or whole milk	1 jalapeño chile, seeded and diced (optional)
Three 4 ounces cans fire-roasted diced green chiles, drained	2 tablespoons chopped fresh cilantro
1 cup nondairy cheese shreds or shredded mozzarella cheese	4 teaspoons extra-virgin olive oil
Salad	4 teaspoons fresh lime juice
1 head green leaf lettuce, shredded	⅛ teaspoon fine sea salt

1. To make the casserole: Pour 1 cup water into the Instant Pot. Butter a 7-cup round heatproof glass dish or coat with nonstick cooking spray and place the dish on a long-handled silicone steam rack. (If you don't have the long-handled rack, use the wire metal steam rack and a homemade sling) 2. In a medium bowl, whisk together the flour and baking powder. Add the eggs and milk and whisk until well blended, forming a batter. Stir in the chiles and ¾ cup of the cheese. 3. Pour the batter into the prepared dish and cover tightly with aluminum foil. Holding the handles of the steam rack, lower the dish into the Instant Pot. 4. Secure the lid and set the Pressure Release to Sealing. Select the Pressure Cook or Manual setting and set the cooking time for 40 minutes at high pressure. (The pot will take about 10 minutes to come up to pressure before the cooking program begins.) 5. When the cooking program ends, let the pressure release naturally for at least 10 minutes, then move the Pressure Release to

Venting to release any remaining steam. Open the pot and, wearing heat-resistant mitts, grasp the handles of the steam rack and lift it out of the pot. Uncover the dish, taking care not to get burned by the steam or to drip condensation onto the casserole. While the casserole is still piping hot, sprinkle the remaining ¼ cup cheese evenly on top. Let the cheese melt for 5 minutes. 6. To make the salad: While the cheese is melting, in a large bowl, combine the lettuce, tomatoes, bell pepper, onion, jalapeño (if using), cilantro, oil, lime juice, and salt. Toss until evenly combined. 7. Cut the casserole into wedges. Serve warm, with the salad on the side.

Per Serving:

calorie: 361 | fat: 22g | protein: 21g | carbs: 23g | sugars: 8g | fiber: 3g | sodium: 421mg

Edamame Falafel with Roasted Vegetables

Prep time: 10 minutes | Cook time: 55 minutes | Serves 2

For the roasted vegetables	1 small onion, chopped
1 cup broccoli florets	1 garlic clove, chopped
1 medium zucchini, sliced	1 tablespoon freshly squeezed lemon juice
½ cup cherry tomatoes, halved	
1½ teaspoons extra-virgin olive oil	2 tablespoons hemp hearts
	1 teaspoon ground cumin
Salt, to season	2 tablespoons oat flour
Freshly ground black pepper, to season	¼ teaspoon salt
	Pinch freshly ground black pepper
Extra-virgin olive oil cooking spray	
	2 tablespoons extra-virgin olive oil, divided
For the falafel	
1 cup frozen shelled edamame, thawed	Prepared hummus, for serving (optional)

To make the roasted vegetables 1. Preheat the oven to 425°F. 2. In a large bowl, toss together the broccoli, zucchini, tomatoes, and olive oil to coat. Season with salt and pepper. 3. Spray a baking sheet with cooking spray. 4. Spread the vegetables evenly atop the sheet. Place the sheet in the preheated oven. Roast for 35 to 40 minutes, stirring every 15 minutes, or until the vegetables are soft and cooked through. 5. Remove from the oven. Set aside. To make the falafel 1. In a food processor, pulse the edamame until coarsely ground. 2. Add the onion, garlic, lemon juice, and hemp hearts. Process until finely ground. Transfer the mixture to a medium bowl. 3. By hand, mix in the cumin, oat flour, salt, and pepper. 4. Roll the dough into 1-inch balls. Flatten slightly. You should have about 12 silver dollar–size patties. 5. In a large skillet set over medium heat, heat 1 tablespoon of olive oil. 6. Add 4 falafel patties to the pan at a time (or as many as will fit without crowding), and cook for about 3 minutes on each side, or until lightly browned. Remove from the pan. Repeat with the remaining 1 tablespoon of olive oil and falafel patties. 7. Serve immediately with the roasted vegetables and hummus (if using) and enjoy!

Per Serving:

calories: 316 | fat: 22g | protein: 12g | carbs: 21g | sugars: 4g | fiber: 6g | sodium: 649mg

Tofu and Bean Chili

Prep time: 10 minutes | Cook time 30 minutes | Serves 4

1 (15 ounces) can low-sodium dark red kidney beans, drained and rinsed, divided
2 (15 ounces) cans no-salt-added diced tomatoes
1½ cups low-sodium vegetable broth
½ teaspoon chili powder
½ teaspoon ground cumin
½ teaspoon garlic powder
½ teaspoon dried oregano
¼ teaspoon onion powder
¼ teaspoon salt
8 ounces extra-firm tofu

1. In a small bowl, mash ⅓ of the beans with a fork. 2. Put the mashed beans, the remaining whole beans, and the diced tomatoes with their juices in a large stockpot. 3. Add the broth, chili powder, cumin, garlic powder, dried oregano, onion powder, and salt. Simmer over medium-high heat for 15 minutes. 4. Press the tofu between 3 or 4 layers of paper towels to squeeze out any excess moisture. 5. Crumble the tofu into the stockpot and stir. Simmer for another 10 to 15 minutes.

Per Serving:

calories: 207 | fat: 5g | protein: 15g | carbs: 31g | sugars: 11g | fiber: 12g | sodium: 376mg

Soybeans with Plums and Peppers

Prep time: 15 minutes | Cook time: 40 minutes | Serves 2

2 medium purple plums
1 tablespoon extra-virgin olive oil
1 medium onion, chopped
1 small yellow bell pepper, chopped
1 small red bell pepper, chopped
1 garlic clove, chopped
2 whole cloves
2 teaspoons ground cumin
½ cup minced fresh cilantro leaves
2 teaspoons freshly squeezed lemon juice
½ teaspoon liquid stevia
1 cup cooked black soybeans

1. Fill a deep pot with water and bring to a boil over high heat. 2. Add the plums. Boil for 30 seconds to loosen their skins. With a slotted spoon, remove the plums. Set aside to cool. 3. In a large skillet set over low heat, heat the olive oil. 4. Add the onion, yellow bell pepper, red bell pepper, garlic, whole cloves, cumin, and cilantro. Cook for 5 to 10 minutes, stirring frequently, until the onion softens. 5. Peel the plums. Remove the pits and chop the fruit. 6. Add the plum, lemon juice, and stevia to the onions and peppers. 7. Stir in the black soybeans. Cover and cook for about 30 minutes, or until the peppers are soft, stirring frequently to prevent sticking. 8. Remove the 2 whole cloves. Serve hot or chilled and enjoy!

Per Serving:

calories: 255 | fat: 5g | protein: 10g | carbs: 46g | sugars: 14g | fiber: 11g | sodium: 22mg

Chickpea and Tofu Bolognese

Prep time: 5 minutes | Cook time: 25 minutes | Serves 4

1 (3 to 4 pounds) spaghetti squash
½ teaspoon ground cumin
1 cup no-sugar-added spaghetti sauce
1 (15 ounces) can low-sodium chickpeas, drained and rinsed
6 ounces extra-firm tofu

1. Preheat the oven to 400°F. 2. Cut the squash in half lengthwise. Scoop out the seeds and discard. 3. Season both halves of the squash with the cumin, and place them on a baking sheet cut-side down. Roast for 25 minutes. 4. Meanwhile, heat a medium saucepan over low heat, and pour in the spaghetti sauce and chickpeas. 5. Press the tofu between two layers of paper towels, and gently squeeze out any excess water. 6. Crumble the tofu into the sauce and cook for 15 minutes. 7. Remove the squash from the oven, and comb through the flesh of each half with a fork to make thin strands. 8. Divide the "spaghetti" into four portions, and top each portion with one-quarter of the sauce.

Per Serving:

calories: 221 | fat: 6g | protein: 12g | carbs: 32g | sugars: 6g | fiber: 8g | sodium: 405mg

Orange Tofu

Prep time: 10 minutes | Cook time: 20 minutes | Serves 4

⅓ cup freshly squeezed orange juice (zest orange first; see orange zest ingredient below)
1 tablespoon tamari
1 tablespoon tahini
½ tablespoon coconut nectar or pure maple syrup
2 tablespoons apple cider vinegar
½ tablespoon freshly grated ginger
1 large clove garlic, grated
½–1 teaspoon orange zest
¼ teaspoon sea salt
Few pinches of crushed red-pepper flakes (optional)
1 package (12 ounces) extra-firm tofu, sliced into ¼"–½" thick squares and patted to remove excess moisture

1. Preheat the oven to 400°F. 2. In a small bowl, combine the orange juice, tamari, tahini, nectar or syrup, vinegar, ginger, garlic, orange zest, salt, and red-pepper flakes (if using). Whisk until well combined. Pour the sauce into an 8" x 12" baking dish. Add the tofu and turn to coat both sides. Bake for 20 minutes. Add salt to taste.

Per Serving:

calorie: 122 | fat: 7g | protein: 10g | carbs: 7g | sugars: 4g | fiber: 1g | sodium: 410mg

Italian Tofu with Mushrooms and Peppers

Prep time: 5 minutes | Cook time: 10 minutes | Serves 2

1 teaspoon extra-virgin olive oil

¼ cup chopped bell pepper, any color

¼ cup chopped onions

1 garlic clove, minced

8 ounces firm tofu, drained and rinsed

½ cup sliced fresh button mushrooms

1 portobello mushroom cap, chopped

1 tablespoon balsamic vinegar

1 teaspoon dried basil

Salt, to season

Freshly ground black pepper, to season

1. In a medium skillet set over medium heat, heat the olive oil. 2. Add the bell pepper, onions, and garlic. Sauté for 5 minutes, or until soft. 3. Add the tofu, button mushrooms, and portobello mushrooms, tossing and stirring. Reduce the heat to low. 4. Stir in the balsamic vinegar and basil. Season with salt and pepper. Simmer for 2 minutes. 5. Enjoy!

Per Serving:

calories: 142 | fat: 8g | protein: 13g | carbs: 9g | sugars: 4g | fiber: 2g | sodium: 326mg

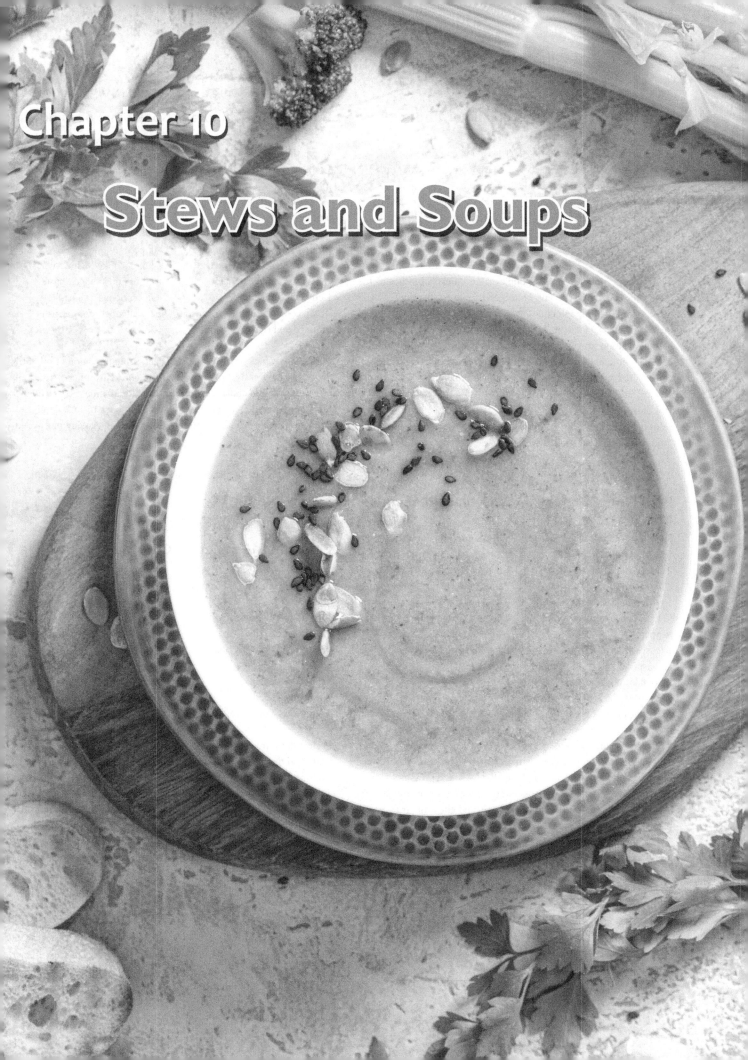

Chapter 10
Stews and Soups

Spanish Black Bean Soup

Prep time: 5 minutes | Cook time: 1 hour 10 minutes | Serves 6

1½ cups plus 2 teaspoons low-sodium chicken broth, divided
1 teaspoon extra-virgin olive oil
3 garlic cloves, minced
1 yellow onion, minced
1 teaspoon minced fresh oregano
1 teaspoon cumin
1 teaspoon chili powder or ½ teaspoon cayenne pepper
1 red bell pepper, chopped
1 carrot, coarsely chopped
3 cups cooked black beans
½ cup dry red wine

1. In a large pot, heat 2 teaspoons of the chicken broth and the olive oil. Add the garlic and onion, and sauté for 3 minutes. Add the oregano, cumin, and chili powder; stir for another minute. Add the red pepper and carrot. 2. Puree 1½ cups of the black beans in a blender or food processor. Add the pureed beans, the remaining 1½ cups of whole black beans, the remaining 1½ cups of chicken broth, and the red wine to the stockpot. Simmer 1 hour. 3. Taste before serving; add additional spices if you like.

Per Serving:

calories: 160 | fat: 3g | protein: 9g | carbs: 25g | sugars: 1g | fiber: 8g | sodium: 48mg

Creamy Sweet Potato Soup

Prep time: 15 minutes | Cook time: 10 minutes | Serves 6

2 tablespoons avocado oil
1 small onion, chopped
2 celery stalks, chopped
2 teaspoons minced garlic
1 teaspoon kosher salt
½ teaspoon freshly ground black pepper
1 teaspoon ground turmeric
½ teaspoon ground cinnamon
2 pounds sweet potatoes, peeled
and cut into 1-inch cubes
3 cups Vegetable Broth or Chicken Bone Broth
Plain Greek yogurt, to garnish (optional)
Chopped fresh parsley, to garnish (optional)
Pumpkin seeds (pepitas), to garnish (optional)

1. Set the electric pressure cooker to the Sauté setting. When the pot is hot, pour in the avocado oil. 2. Sauté the onion and celery for 3 to 5 minutes or until the vegetables begin to soften. 3. Stir in the garlic, salt, pepper, turmeric, and cinnamon. Hit Cancel. 4. Stir in the sweet potatoes and broth. 5. Close and lock the lid of the pressure cooker. Set the valve to sealing. 6. Cook on high pressure for 10 minutes. 7. When the cooking is complete, hit Cancel and allow the pressure to release naturally. 8. Once the pin drops, unlock and remove the lid. 9. Use an immersion blender to purée the soup right in the pot. If you don't have an immersion blender, transfer the soup to a blender or food processor and purée. (Follow the instructions that came with your machine for blending hot foods.) 10. Spoon into bowls and serve topped with Greek yogurt, parsley, and/or pumpkin seeds (if using).

Per Serving:

calories: 175 | fat: 5g | protein: 5g | carbs: 29g | sugars: 4g | fiber: 4g | sodium: 706mg

Hearty Italian Minestrone

Prep time: 10 minutes | Cook time: 50 minutes | Serves 8

½ cup sliced onion
1 tablespoon extra-virgin olive oil
4 cups low-sodium chicken broth
¾ cup diced carrot
½ cup diced potato (with skin)
2 cups sliced cabbage or coarsely chopped spinach
1 cup diced zucchini
½ cup cooked garbanzo beans (drained and rinsed, if canned)
½ cup cooked navy beans (drained and rinsed, if canned)
One 14½-ounce can low-sodium tomatoes, with liquid
½ cup diced celery
2 tablespoons fresh basil, finely chopped
½ cup uncooked whole-wheat rotini or other shaped pasta
2 tablespoons fresh parsley, finely chopped, for garnish

1. In a large stockpot over medium heat, sauté the onion in oil until the onion is slightly browned. Add the chicken broth, carrot, and potato. Cover and cook over medium heat for 30 minutes. 2. Add the remaining ingredients and cook for an additional 15 to 20 minutes, until the pasta is cooked through. Garnish with parsley and serve hot.

Per Serving:

calories: 101 | fat: 2g | protein: 6g | carbs: 17g | sugars: 4g | fiber: 4g | sodium: 108mg

Minted Sweet Pea Soup

Prep time: 10 minutes | Cook time: 10 minutes | Serves 2 to 4

2 tablespoons extra-virgin olive oil
1 small yellow onion, minced
Pinch kosher salt
Pinch freshly ground black pepper
2 garlic cloves, minced
1 zucchini, diced
4 cups low-sodium vegetable broth
3 cups frozen peas
Juice of 1 lemon
½ cup plain Greek yogurt (optional)
½ cup thinly sliced fresh mint
2 tablespoons chopped pistachios (optional)

1. Heat the extra-virgin olive oil in a medium stockpot over medium heat. Add the onion, salt, and pepper and sauté until translucent. 2. Add the garlic and zucchini and sauté until tender, about 3 minutes. 3. Transfer the vegetables to a blender and puree them with the vegetable broth, peas, and lemon juice. 4. Adjust the seasonings as desired and serve the soup warmed in a saucepan over medium heat or cooled in the refrigerator. To cool it in an ice bath, transfer the soup to a medium bowl and nestle that in a large bowl filled with ice water. 5. Serve with a dollop of optional Greek yogurt (if using) and topped with mint and pistachios (if using). 6. Store the cooled soup in an airtight container in the refrigerator for up to 5 days, with garnishes kept separately.

Per Serving:

calories: 181 | fat: 6g | protein: 8g | carbs: 27g | sugars: 13g | fiber: 6g | sodium: 442mg

Pumpkin and Black Bean Soup

Prep time: 15 minutes | Cook time: 35 minutes | Serves 2

2 teaspoons extra-virgin olive oil	drained and rinsed
1 small onion, finely chopped	1 (8 ounces) can solid-pack pumpkin
1 small red bell pepper, chopped	1 cup almond milk, or soy milk
1 garlic clove, minced	½ cup frozen spinach
1 teaspoon ground cumin	Salt, to season
1 cup low-sodium vegetable broth	Freshly ground black pepper, to season
1 cup diced tomatoes, with juice	Chopped fresh chives, for garnish
1 cup canned black beans,	

1. In a medium pot set over medium heat, heat the olive oil. 2. Stir in the onion and bell pepper. Cook for about 5 minutes, stirring, until the onion softens and turns translucent. 3. Mix in the garlic and cumin. Cook, stirring, for 2 minutes more. 4. Add the vegetable broth, tomatoes, black beans, pumpkin, almond milk, and spinach. Stir to combine. 5. Season with salt and pepper. 6. Bring the soup to a gentle boil. Reduce the heat to low. Simmer, covered, for 25 minutes. 7. Garnish each bowl of soup with chives and enjoy!

Per Serving:

calories: 452 | fat: 16g | protein: 22g | carbs: 60g | sugars: 15g | fiber: 18g | sodium: 457mg

Chicken Brunswick Stew

Prep time: 0 minutes | Cook time: 30 minutes | Serves 6

2 tablespoons extra-virgin olive oil	1 cup low-sodium chicken broth
2 garlic cloves, chopped	1 tablespoon hot sauce (such as Tabasco or Crystal)
1 large yellow onion, diced	1 tablespoon raw apple cider vinegar
2 pounds boneless, skinless chicken (breasts, tenders, or thighs), cut into bite-size pieces	1½ cups frozen corn
1 teaspoon dried thyme	1½ cups frozen baby lima beans
1 teaspoon smoked paprika	One 14½ ounces can fire-roasted diced tomatoes and their liquid
1 teaspoon fine sea salt	2 tablespoons tomato paste
½ teaspoon freshly ground black pepper	Cornbread, for serving

1. Select the Sauté setting on the Instant Pot and heat the oil and garlic for 2 minutes, until the garlic is bubbling but not browned. Add the onion and sauté for 3 minutes, until it begins to soften. Add the chicken and sauté for 3 minutes more, until mostly opaque. The chicken does not have to be cooked through. Add the thyme, paprika, salt, and pepper and sauté for 1 minute more. 2. Stir in the broth, hot sauce, vinegar, corn, and lima beans. Add the diced tomatoes and their liquid in an even layer and dollop the tomato paste on top. Do not stir them in. 3. Secure the lid and set the Pressure Release to Sealing. Press the Cancel button to reset the cooking program, then select the Pressure Cook or Manual setting and set the cooking time for 5 minutes at high pressure. (The pot will take about 15 minutes to come up to pressure before the cooking program begins.) 4. When the cooking program ends, let the pressure release naturally for at least 10 minutes, then move the Pressure Release to Venting to release any remaining steam. Open the pot and stir the stew to mix all of the ingredients. 5. Ladle the stew into bowls and serve hot, with cornbread alongside.

Per Serving:

calories: 349 | fat: 7g | protein: 40g | carbs: 17g | sugars: 7g | fiber: 7g | sodium: 535mg

Tomato and Kale Soup

Prep time: 10 minutes | Cook time: 15 minutes | Serves 4

1 tablespoon extra-virgin olive oil	1 (28-ounce) can crushed tomatoes
1 medium onion, chopped	½ teaspoon dried oregano
2 carrots, finely chopped	¼ teaspoon dried basil
3 garlic cloves, minced	4 cups chopped baby kale leaves
4 cups low-sodium vegetable broth	¼ teaspoon salt

1. In a large pot, heat the oil over medium heat. Add the onion and carrots to the pan. Sauté for 3 to 5 minutes until they begin to soften. Add the garlic and sauté for 30 seconds more, until fragrant. 2. Add the vegetable broth, tomatoes, oregano, and basil to the pot and bring to a boil. Reduce the heat to low and simmer for 5 minutes. 3. Using an immersion blender, purée the soup. 4. Add the kale and simmer for 3 more minutes. Season with the salt. Serve immediately.

Per Serving:

calories: 170 | fat: 5g | protein: 6g | carbs: 31g | sugars: 13g | fiber: 9g | sodium: 600mg

Kickin' Chili

Prep time: 10 minutes | Cook time: 45 minutes | Serves 2

1 tablespoon extra-virgin olive oil	1 (15 ounces) can pinto beans, drained and rinsed
½ cup chopped onions	2 cups water
1 garlic clove, minced	2 teaspoons ground cumin
1 celery stalk, chopped	2 teaspoons chili powder
½ cup chopped bell peppers, any color	½ teaspoon cayenne pepper
1 cup diced tomatoes, undrained	Salt, to season
1 cup frozen broccoli florets	Freshly ground black pepper, to season

1. In a large pot set over medium heat, heat the olive oil. 2. Add the onions. Cook for about 5 minutes, or until tender. 3. Add the garlic. Cook for 2 to 3 minutes, or until lightly browned. 4. Add the celery and bell peppers. Cook for 5 minutes, or until the vegetables are soft. 5. Stir in the tomatoes, broccoli, pinto beans, and water. 6. Add the cumin, chili powder, and cayenne pepper. Season with salt and pepper. Stir to combine. Simmer for 30 minutes, stirring frequently. 7. Serve hot and enjoy!

Per Serving:

calories: 249 | fat: 5g | protein: 14g | carbs: 42g | sugars: 6g | fiber: 13g | sodium: 739mg

French Market Soup

Prep time: 20 minutes | Cook time: 1 hour | Serves 8

2 cups mixed dry beans, washed with stones removed	16-ounce can low-sodium tomatoes
7 cups water	1 large onion, chopped
1 ham hock, all visible fat removed	1 garlic clove, minced
1 teaspoon salt	1 chile, chopped, or 1 teaspoon chili powder
¼ teaspoon pepper	¼ cup lemon juice

1. Combine all ingredients in the inner pot of the Instant Pot. 2. Secure the lid and make sure vent is set to sealing. Using Manual, set the Instant Pot to cook for 60 minutes. 3. When cooking time is over, let the pressure release naturally. When the Instant Pot is ready, unlock the lid, then remove the bone and any hard or fatty pieces. Pull the meat off the bone and chop into small pieces. Add the ham back into the Instant Pot.

Per Serving:
calories: 191 | fat: 4g | protein: 12g | carbs: 29g | sugars: 5g | fiber: 7g | sodium: 488mg

Pasta e Fagioli with Ground Beef

Prep time: 0 minutes | Cook time: 30 minutes | Serves 8

2 tablespoons extra-virgin olive oil	1¼ cups chickpea-based elbow pasta or whole-wheat elbow pasta
4 garlic cloves, minced	
1 yellow onion, diced	1½ cups drained cooked kidney beans, or one 15-ounce can kidney beans, rinsed and drained
2 large carrots, diced	
4 celery stalks, diced	
1½ pounds 95 percent extra-lean ground beef	
4 cups low-sodium vegetable broth	One 28-ounce can whole San Marzano tomatoes and their liquid
2 teaspoons Italian seasoning	
½ teaspoon freshly ground black pepper	2 tablespoons chopped fresh flat-leaf parsley

1. Select the Sauté setting on the Instant Pot and heat the oil and garlic for 2 minutes, until the garlic is bubbling but not browned. Add the onion, carrots, and celery and sauté for 5 minutes, until the onion begins to soften. Add the beef and sauté, using a wooden spoon or spatula to break up the meat as it cooks, for 5 minutes; it's fine if some streaks of pink remain, the beef does not need to be cooked through. 2. Stir in the broth, Italian seasoning, pepper, and pasta, making sure all of the pasta is submerged in the liquid. Add the beans and stir to mix. Add the tomatoes and their liquid, crushing the tomatoes with your hands as you add them to the pot. Do not stir them in. 3. Secure the lid and set the Pressure Release to Sealing. Press the Cancel button to reset the cooking program, then select the Pressure Cook or Manual setting and set the cooking time for 2 minutes at low pressure. (The pot will take about 15 minutes to come up to pressure before the cooking program begins.) 4. When the cooking program ends, let the pressure release naturally for 10 minutes, then move the Pressure Release to Venting to release any remaining steam. Open the pot and stir the soup to mix all of the ingredients. 5. Ladle the soup into bowls, sprinkle with the parsley, and serve right away.

Per Serving:
calories: 278 | fat: 9g | protein: 26g | carbs: 25g | sugars: 4g | fiber: 6g | sodium: 624mg

African Peanut Stew

Prep time: 10 minutes | Cook time: 35 minutes | Serves 2

3 cups low-sodium vegetable broth	½ cup unsalted natural peanut butter
1 small onion, chopped	2 tablespoons tomato paste
1 small red bell pepper, chopped	1 bunch kale, thoroughly washed, deveined, and chopped (about 2½ cups)
1 medium carrot, chopped	
1 tablespoon minced fresh ginger	
2 garlic cloves, minced	Freshly ground black pepper, to season
¼ teaspoon salt, plus more to season	2 scallions, chopped

1. In a medium pot set over medium-low heat, bring the vegetable broth to a boil. 2. Add the onion, bell pepper, carrot, ginger, garlic, and salt. Cook for 20 minutes. 3. In a medium, heat-safe mixing bowl, stir together the peanut butter and tomato paste. 4. Transfer 1 cup of the hot vegetable broth to the bowl. Whisk until smooth. Pour the peanut butter mixture back into the soup. Mix well to combine. 5. Stir in the kale. Season with salt and pepper. Simmer for about 15 minutes more, stirring frequently. 6. Top with the scallions and enjoy!

Per Serving:
calories: 565 | fat: 36g | protein: 24g | carbs: 51g | sugars: 26g | fiber: 12g | sodium: 580mg

Nancy's Vegetable Beef Soup

Prep time: 25 minutes | Cook time: 8 hours | Serves 8

2 pounds roast, cubed, or 2 pounds stewing meat	stewed tomatoes
15 ounces can corn	5 teaspoons salt-free beef bouillon powder
15 ounces can green beans	Tabasco, to taste
1 pound bag frozen peas	½ teaspoons salt
40 ounces can no-added-salt	

1. Combine all ingredients in the Instant Pot. Do not drain vegetables. 2. Add water to fill inner pot only to the fill line. 3. Secure the lid, or use the glass lid and set the Instant Pot on Slow Cook mode, Low for 8 hours, or until meat is tender and vegetables are soft.

Per Serving:
calories: 229 | fat: 5g | protein: 23g | carbs: 24g | sugars: 10g | fiber: 6g | sodium: 545mg

Golden Chicken Soup

Prep time: 10 minutes | Cook time: 20 minutes | Serves 4 to 6

1 tablespoon extra-virgin olive oil	6 cups low-sodium chicken broth
1 yellow onion, chopped	3 (5 to 6 ounces) boneless, skinless chicken breasts
2 teaspoons garlic powder	
1 tablespoon ginger powder	4 celery stalks, cut into ¼-inch-thick slices
2 teaspoons turmeric	
½ teaspoon freshly ground black pepper	1 fennel bulb, thinly sliced

1. Heat the extra-virgin olive oil in a large stockpot over medium heat. Sauté the onion until translucent, about 3 minutes. Add the garlic powder, ginger powder, turmeric, black pepper, and chicken broth. 2. Bring to a boil, then carefully add the chicken, celery, and fennel. Reduce the heat to medium-low, cover, and simmer until the internal temperature of the chicken is 160°F, 5 to 10 minutes. 3. Remove the chicken breasts and allow them to cool for 5 minutes while the soup keeps simmering. 4. Shred the chicken using two forks and return it to the stockpot. Heat the soup for about 1 minute and adjust the seasonings as desired. 5. Store the cooled soup in an airtight container in the refrigerator for 3 to 5 days.

Per Serving:

calories: 107 | fat: 4g | protein: 10g | carbs: 10g | sugars: 3g | fiber: 2g | sodium: 370mg

Hodgepodge Stew

Prep time: 10 minutes | Cook time: 25 minutes | Serves 4

3 tablespoons water	flour
2 cups roughly chopped onion	2 cups vegetable stock
2 to 2½ cups cauliflower florets	3 cups cubed potatoes (can substitute sweet potatoes)
1½ cups thickly sliced carrots	
1 teaspoon dried thyme leaves	1 can (15 ounces) kidney beans, drained and rinsed
1 teaspoon dried savory or rosemary leaves (or ½ teaspoon each)	
	1½ cups low-fat nondairy milk
1 teaspoon mustard seeds	1 cup chopped green beans or frozen green peas
½ teaspoon dill seed (optional)	
¼ teaspoon sea salt	2 tablespoons nutritional yeast (optional)
3 tablespoons spelt or other	

1. In a large pot over medium-high heat, combine the water, onion, cauliflower, carrots, thyme, savory or rosemary, mustard seeds, dill (if using), and salt. Cook for 3 to 4 minutes, stirring a few times. Add the flour and stir frequently for another few minutes, to help cook out the raw flavor of the flour. Add a splash of the vegetable stock if needed to prevent sticking. Add the remainder of the stock gradually, starting with ¼ to ½ cup and stirring it into the flour steadily, allowing the flour and stock to thicken together. Let the mixture bubble, and then continue adding the stock. Add the potatoes and beans, and let the mixture come to a boil. Reduce the heat to medium-low, cover the pot, and cook for 15 minutes, or until the

potatoes are tender when pierced. Add the milk, green beans or peas, and yeast (if using). Heat through for 4 to 5 minutes, then serve.

Per Serving:

calorie: 250 | fat: 2g | protein: 10g | carbs: 51g | sugars: 11g | fiber: 9g | sodium: 558mg

Chicken Rice Soup

Prep time: 10 minutes | Cook time: 10 minutes | Serves 8

1 teaspoon vegetable oil	chicken breasts, cut into ¾" cubes
2 ribs celery, chopped in ½"-thick pieces	
	5¼ cups fat-free, low-sodium chicken broth
1 medium onion, chopped	
1 cup wild rice, uncooked	2 teaspoons dried thyme leaves
½ cup long-grain rice, uncooked	¼ teaspoon red pepper flakes
1 pound boneless skinless	

1. Using the Sauté function on the Instant Pot, heat the teaspoon of vegetable oil. Sauté the celery and onion until the onions are slightly translucent (3–5 minutes). Once cooked, press Cancel. 2. Add the remaining ingredients to the inner pot. 3. Secure the lid and make sure the vent is set to sealing. Using the Manual function, set the time to 10 minutes. 4. When cook time is over, let the pressure release naturally for 10 minutes, then perform a quick release.

Per Serving:

calories: 160 | fat: 2g | protein: 16g | carbs: 18g | sugars: 2g | fiber: 1g | sodium: 375mg

Lentil Stew

Prep time: 10 minutes | Cook time: 30 minutes | Serves 2

½ cup dry lentils, picked through, debris removed, rinsed and drained	2 medium tomatoes, diced
	1 celery stalk, chopped
	1 tablespoon extra-virgin olive oil
2½ cups water	
1 bay leaf	1 medium onion, diced
2 teaspoons dried tarragon	1 cup frozen spinach
2 teaspoons dried thyme	Salt, to season
2 garlic cloves, minced	Freshly ground black pepper, to season
2 medium carrots, chopped	

1. In a soup pot set over high heat, stir together the lentils, water, bay leaf, tarragon, thyme, and garlic. 2. Add the carrots, tomatoes, and celery. Cover. Bring to a boil. Reduce the heat to low and stir the soup. Simmer for 15 to 20 minutes, covered, or until the lentils are tender. 3. While the vegetables simmer, place a skillet over medium heat. Add the olive oil and onion. Sauté for about 10 minutes, or until browned. Remove the skillet from the heat. 4. When the lentils are tender, remove and discard the bay leaf. Add the cooked onion and the spinach to the soup. Heat for 5 to 10 minutes more, or until the spinach is cooked. 5. Season with salt and pepper. 6. Enjoy immediately.

Per Serving:

calories: 214 | fat: 7g | protein: 10g | carbs: 31g | sugars: 10g | fiber: 11g | sodium: 871mg

Cauliflower Chili

Prep time: 10 minutes | Cook time: 35 minutes | Serves 5

2 cups thickly sliced carrot	⅛ teaspoon allspice
½ large or 1 full small head cauliflower	¼ teaspoon crushed red-pepper flakes (or to taste)
4 or 5 cloves garlic, minced	1 can (28 ounces) crushed tomatoes
1 tablespoon balsamic vinegar	1 can (15 ounces) pinto beans, rinsed and drained
1½ cups diced onion	
1 teaspoon sea salt	1 can (15 ounces) kidney beans or black beans, rinsed and drained
1½ tablespoons mild chili powder	
1 tablespoon cocoa powder	½ cup water
2 teaspoons ground cumin	Lime wedges
2 teaspoons dried oregano	

1. In a food processor, combine the carrot, cauliflower, and garlic, and pulse until finely minced. (Alternatively, you could mince by hand.) In a large pot over medium heat, combine the vinegar, onion, salt, chili powder, cocoa, cumin, oregano, allspice, and red-pepper flakes. Cook for 3 to 4 minutes, stirring occasionally. Add the minced carrot, cauliflower, and garlic, and cook for 5 to 6 minutes, stirring occasionally. Add the tomatoes, pinto and kidney beans, and water, and stir to combine. Increase the heat to high to bring to a boil. Reduce the heat to low, cover, and simmer for 25 minutes. Taste, and season as desired. Serve with lime wedges.

Per Serving:

calorie: 237 | fat: 3g | protein: 13g | carbs: 45g | sugars: 13g | fiber: 15g | sodium: 1036mg

Chicken Noodle Soup

Prep time: 15 minutes | Cook time: 20 minutes | Serves 12

2 tablespoons avocado oil	3 pounds bone-in chicken breasts (about 3)
1 medium onion, chopped	
3 celery stalks, chopped	4 cups Chicken Bone Broth or low-sodium store-bought chicken broth
1 teaspoon kosher salt	
¼ teaspoon freshly ground black pepper	
	4 cups water
2 teaspoons minced garlic	2 tablespoons soy sauce
5 large carrots, peeled and cut into ¼-inch-thick rounds	6 ounces whole grain wide egg noodles

1. Set the electric pressure cooker to the Sauté setting. When the pot is hot, pour in the avocado oil. 2. Sauté the onion, celery, salt, and pepper for 3 to 5 minutes or until the vegetables begin to soften. 3. Add the garlic and carrots, and stir to mix well. Hit Cancel. 4. Add the chicken to the pot, meat-side down. Add the broth, water, and soy sauce. Close and lock the lid of the pressure cooker. Set the valve to sealing. 5. Cook on high pressure for 20 minutes. 6. When the cooking is complete, hit Cancel and quick release the pressure. Unlock and remove the lid. 7. Using tongs, remove the chicken breasts to a cutting board. Hit Sauté/More and bring the soup to a boil. 8. Add the noodles and cook for 4 to 5 minutes or until the noodles are al dente. 9. While the noodles are cooking, use two forks to shred the chicken. Add the meat back to the pot and save the bones to make more bone broth. 10. Season with additional pepper, if desired, and serve.

Per Serving:

calories: 294 | fat: 14g | protein: 27g | carbs: 15g | sugars: 3g | fiber: 3g | sodium: 640mg

Herbed Chicken Stew with Noodles

Prep time: 10 minutes | Cook time: 40 minutes | Serves 8

1 tablespoon extra-virgin olive oil	broth
	1 cup dry white wine
1 onion, chopped	1 tablespoon chopped fresh thyme (or 1 teaspoon dried)
2 garlic cloves, minced	
1 pound boneless, skinless chicken breast, cubed	4 cups cooked egg noodles, hot (from 1/2 pound dry egg noodles)
2 tablespoons flour	
3 cups low-sodium chicken	½ cup minced parsley

1. In a large saucepan, heat the oil and sauté the onion and garlic for about 5 minutes. Add the chicken cubes, and sauté until the chicken is cooked (about 10 minutes). 2. Sprinkle the flour over the chicken. Add the chicken broth, wine, and thyme. Bring to a boil, and then lower the heat and simmer for 30 minutes. 3. Toss together the noodles and the parsley in a large bowl. Pour the stew over the noodles and serve.

Per Serving:

calories: 285 | fat: 9g | protein: 14g | carbs: 37g | sugars: 4g | fiber: 2g | sodium: 419mg

Golden Lentil—Pea Soup

Prep time: 10 minutes | Cook time: 50 minutes | Serves 6

1 cup diced onion	potato (or 2 cups chopped sweet potato and 2 cups chopped carrot)
1 cup chopped celery	
1 tablespoon smoked paprika	
1 teaspoon dried rosemary	1½ cups dried red lentils
1 teaspoon ground cumin	1 cup dried yellow split peas
¼ teaspoon allspice	2 cups vegetable broth
¼ teaspoon sea salt	1½ tablespoons apple cider vinegar
2–3 tablespoons + 4 cups water	
4 cups chopped yellow sweet	

1. In a large soup pot over medium-high heat, combine the onion, celery, paprika, rosemary, cumin, allspice, salt, and 2 to 3 tablespoons of the water, and stir. Cook for 8 to 9 minutes, then add the potato, lentils, split peas, broth, and the remaining 4 cups of water. Stir to combine. Increase the heat to high to bring to a boil. Reduce the heat to low, cover, and simmer for 40 to 45 minutes, or until the peas are completely softened. Stir in the apple cider vinegar, season with additional salt and pepper if desired, and serve.

Per Serving:

calorie: 340 | fat: 1g | protein: 21g | carbs: 64g | sugars: 8g | fiber: 20g | sodium: 363mg

Beef and Mushroom Barley Soup

Prep time: 10 minutes | Cook time: 1 hour 20 minutes | Serves 6

1 pound beef stew meat, cubed	2 carrots, chopped
¼ teaspoon salt	3 celery stalks, chopped
¼ teaspoon freshly ground black pepper	6 garlic cloves, minced
	½ teaspoon dried thyme
1 tablespoon extra-virgin olive oil	4 cups low-sodium beef broth
	1 cup water
8 ounces sliced mushrooms	½ cup pearl barley
1 onion, chopped	

1. Season the meat with the salt and pepper. 2. In an Instant Pot, heat the oil over high heat. Add the meat and brown on all sides. Remove the meat from the pot and set aside. 3. Add the mushrooms to the pot and cook for 1 to 2 minutes, until they begin to soften. Remove the mushrooms and set aside with the meat. 4. Add the onion, carrots, and celery to the pot. Sauté for 3 to 4 minutes until the vegetables begin to soften. Add the garlic and continue to cook until fragrant, about 30 seconds longer. 5. Return the meat and mushrooms to the pot, then add the thyme, beef broth, and water. Set the pressure to high and cook for 15 minutes. Let the pressure release naturally. 6. Open the Instant Pot and add the barley. Use the slow cooker function on the Instant Pot, affix the lid (vent open), and continue to cook for 1 hour until the barley is cooked through and tender. Serve.

Per Serving:

calories: 245 | fat: 9g | protein: 21g | carbs: 19g | sugars: 3g | fiber: 4g | sodium: 516mg

Black Bean Soup with Sweet Potatoes

Prep time: 10 minutes | Cook time: 30 minutes | Serves 4

1 tablespoon balsamic vinegar	4 medium-large cloves garlic, minced or grated
1½ to 1¾ cups chopped onion	
1½ cups combination of chopped red and green bell peppers	2 tablespoons tomato paste
	2 tablespoons freshly squeezed lime juice
1 teaspoon sea salt	½ to 1 teaspoon pure maple syrup
Freshly ground black pepper to taste	
2 teaspoons cumin seeds	4½ cups (about 3 cans, 15 ounces each) black beans, drained and rinsed
2 teaspoons dried oregano leaves	
	1 bay leaf
Rounded ¼ teaspoon allspice	1½ cups ½" cubes yellow sweet potato (can substitute white potato)
¼ teaspoon red-pepper flakes, or to taste	
1 to 4 tablespoons + 3 cups water	Chopped cilantro (optional)
	Extra lime wedges (optional)

1. In a large pot over medium-high heat, combine the vinegar, onion, bell peppers, salt, black pepper, cumin seeds, oregano, allspice, and red-pepper flakes. Cook for 5 to 7 minutes, or until the onions and red peppers start to soften. Add 1 to 2 tablespoons of water if needed to keep the vegetables from sticking. Add the garlic and stir. Cover, reduce the heat to medium, and cook for another few minutes, until the garlic is softened. If anything is sticking or burning, add another 1 to 2 tablespoons of water. When the garlic is soft, add the tomato paste, lime juice, ½ teaspoon of the syrup, 3½ cups of the beans, and the remaining 3 cups water. Use an immersion blender to puree the soup until it's fairly smooth. Add the bay leaf and sweet potato, increase the heat to high to bring to a boil, then reduce the heat to low and simmer for 20 to 30 minutes. Add the remaining 1 cup black beans. Taste, and add the remaining ½ teaspoon syrup, if desired. Stir, simmer for another few minutes, then serve, seasoning to taste and topping with the cilantro (if using) and lime wedges (if using).

Per Serving:

calorie: 368 | fat: 2g | protein: 19g | carbs: 73g | sugars: 10g | fiber: 24g | sodium: 1049mg

Minestrone with Parmigiano-Reggiano

Prep time: 25 minutes | Cook time: 3 to 8 hours | Serves 8

2 tablespoons extra-virgin olive oil	cabbage, cut into small pieces
	8 ounces (227 g) green beans, ends snipped, cut into 1-inch pieces
3 cloves garlic, minced	
1 cup coarsely chopped sweet onion	
	1 medium head cauliflower, cut into florets
1 cup coarsely chopped carrots	
1 cup coarsely chopped celery	Rind from Parmigiano-Reggiano cheese, cut into ½-inch pieces, plus ½ to 1 cup finely grated Parmigiano-Reggiano cheese, for garnish
1 tablespoon finely chopped fresh rosemary	
1 (14- to 15-ounce / 397- to 425-g) can plum tomatoes, with their juice	
	2 cups vegetable broth
¼ cup dry white wine	1 teaspoon salt
2 medium zucchini, cut into ½-inch rounds	½ teaspoon freshly ground black pepper
1 (14- to 15-ounce / 397- to 425-g) can small white beans, drained and rinsed	8 ounces (227 g) cooked small pasta (shells, ditalini, or other short tubular pasta)
1 head escarole or Savoy	

1. Heat the oil in a large skillet over medium-high heat. Add the garlic, onion, carrots, celery, and rosemary and sauté until the vegetables begin to soften, 4 to 5 minutes. 2. Add the tomatoes and wine and allow some of the liquid to evaporate in the pan. 3. Transfer the contents of the skillet to the insert of a 5- to 7-quart slow cooker. Add the zucchini, white beans, cabbage, green beans, cauliflower, Parmigiano-Reggiano rind, broth, salt, and pepper. 4. Cover the slow cooker and cook on high for 3 to 4 hours or on low for 6 to 8 hours. 5. Stir in the cooked pasta at the end of the cooking time, cover, and set on warm until ready to serve. Serve the soup garnished with the grated Parmigiano-Reggiano.

Per Serving:

calories: 224 | fat: 5g | protein: 9g | carbs: 40g | sugars: 11g | fiber: g | sodium: 552mg

Buttercup Squash Soup

Prep time: 15 minutes | Cook time: 10 minutes | Serves 6

2 tablespoons extra-virgin olive oil
1 medium onion, chopped
4 to 5 cups Vegetable Broth or Chicken Bone Broth
1½ pounds buttercup squash,

peeled, seeded, and cut into 1-inch chunks
½ teaspoon kosher salt
¼ teaspoon ground white pepper
Whole nutmeg, for grating

1. Set the electric pressure cooker to the Sauté setting. When the pot is hot, pour in the olive oil. 2. Add the onion and sauté for 3 to 5 minutes, until it begins to soften. Hit Cancel. 3. Add the broth, squash, salt, and pepper to the pot and stir. (If you want a thicker soup, use 4 cups of broth. If you want a thinner, drinkable soup, use 5 cups.) 4. Close and lock the lid of the pressure cooker. Set the valve to sealing. 5. Cook on high pressure for 10 minutes. 6. When the cooking is complete, hit Cancel and allow the pressure to release naturally. 7. Once the pin drops, unlock and remove the lid. 8. Use an immersion blender to purée the soup right in the pot. If you don't have an immersion blender, transfer the soup to a blender or food processor and purée. (Follow the instructions that came with your machine for blending hot foods.) 9. Pour the soup into serving bowls and grate nutmeg on top.

Per Serving:
calories: 320 | fat: 16g | protein: 36g | carbs: 7g | sugars: 3g | fiber: 2g | sodium: 856mg

Ham and Potato Chowder

Prep time: 25 minutes | Cook time: 8 hour s | Serves 5

5-ounce package scalloped potatoes
Sauce mix from potato package
1 cup extra-lean, reduced-sodium, cooked ham, cut into narrow strips
4 teaspoons sodium-free

bouillon powder
4 cups water
1 cup chopped celery
⅓ cup chopped onions
Pepper to taste
2 cups fat-free half-and-half
⅓ cup flour

1. Combine potatoes, sauce mix, ham, bouillon powder, water, celery, onions, and pepper in the inner pot of the Instant Pot. 2. Secure the lid and cook using the Slow Cook function on low for 7 hours. 3. Combine half-and-half and flour. Remove the lid and gradually add to the inner pot, blending well. 4. Secure the lid once more and cook on the low Slow Cook function for up to 1 hour more, stirring occasionally until thickened.

Per Serving:
calories: 241 | fat: 3g | protein: 11g | carbs: 41g | sugars: 8g | fiber: 3g | sodium: 836mg

Pasta e Fagioli

Prep time: 10 minutes | Cook time: 25 minutes | Serves 12

1 tablespoon extra-virgin olive oil
1 large onion, chopped
3 cloves garlic, crushed
2 medium carrots, sliced
2 medium zucchini, sliced
2 tablespoons finely chopped fresh basil
2 teaspoons finely chopped

fresh oregano
Two 14½-ounce cans unsalted tomatoes with liquid
Two 15-ounce cans low-sodium white cannellini or navy beans, drained and rinsed
¾ pound whole-wheat uncooked rigatoni or shell pasta

1. In a large saucepan, heat the oil and sauté the onion and garlic for 5 minutes. 2. Add the carrots, zucchini, basil, oregano, tomatoes with their liquid, and beans. Cook until the vegetables are just tender, about 15–17 minutes. 3. In a separate saucepan, cook the pasta according to package directions (without adding salt). Add the pasta to the soup, and mix thoroughly. Serve warm with crusty bread.

Per Serving:
calories: 84 | fat: 1g | protein: 4g | carbs: 16g | sugars: 1g | fiber: 3g | sodium: 68mg

Freshened-Up French Onion Soup

Prep time: 15 minutes | Cook time: 30 minutes | Serves 2

1 tablespoon extra-virgin olive oil
2 medium onions, sliced
2 cups low-sodium beef broth
1 (8-ounce) can chickpeas, drained and rinsed

½ teaspoon dried thyme
Salt
Freshly ground black pepper
4 slices nonfat Swiss deli-style cheese

1. In a medium soup pot set over medium-low heat, heat the olive oil. 2. Add the onions. Stir to coat them in oil. Cook for about 10 minutes, or until golden brown. 3. Add the beef broth, chickpeas, and thyme. Bring to a simmer. 4. Taste the broth. Season with salt and pepper. Cook for 10 minutes more. 5. Preheat the broiler to high. 6. Ladle the soup into 2 ovenproof soup bowls. 7. Top each with 2 slices of Swiss cheese. Place the bowls on a baking sheet. Carefully transfer the sheet to the preheated oven. Melt the cheese under the broiler for 2 minutes. Alternately, you can melt the cheese in the microwave (in microwave-safe bowls) on high in 30-second intervals until melted. 8. Enjoy immediately.

Per Serving:
calories: 278 | fat: 14g | protein: 15g | carbs: 29g | sugars: 3g | fiber: 2g | sodium: 804mg

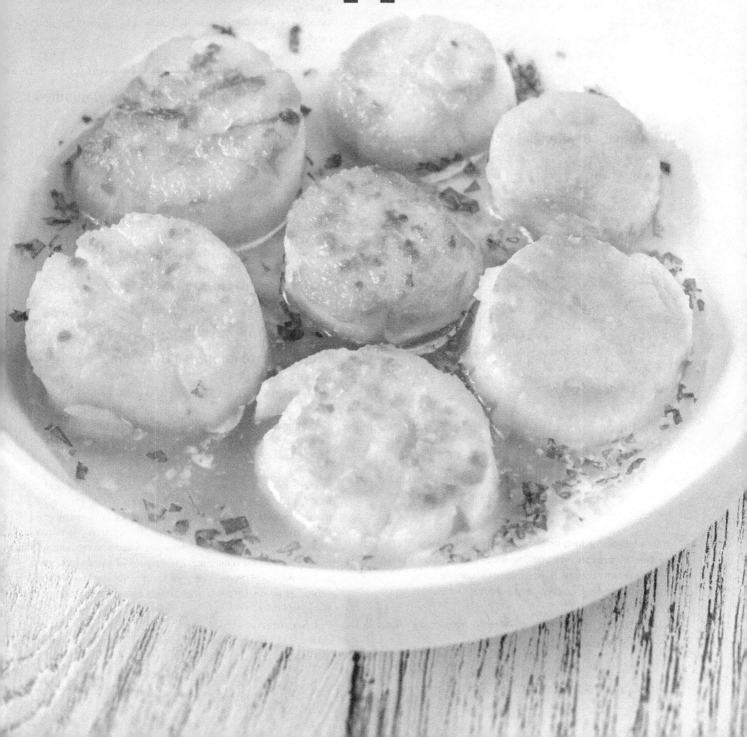

Chapter 11
Snacks and Appetizers

Spinach and Artichoke Dip

Prep time: 5 minutes | Cook time: 4 minutes | Serves 11

8 ounces low-fat cream cheese
10-ounce box frozen spinach
½ cup no-sodium chicken broth
14-ounce can artichoke hearts, drained
½ cup low-fat sour cream
½ cup low-fat mayo

3 cloves of garlic, minced
1 teaspoon onion powder
16 ounces reduced-fat shredded Parmesan cheese
8 ounces reduced-fat shredded mozzarella

1. Put all ingredients in the inner pot of the Instant Pot, except the Parmesan cheese and the mozzarella cheese. 2. Secure the lid and set vent to sealing. Place on Manual high pressure for 4 minutes. 3. Do a quick release of steam. 4. Immediately stir in the cheeses.

Per Serving:
calories: 288 | fat: 18g | protein: 19g | carbs: 15g | sugars: 3g | fiber: 3g | sodium: 1007mg

Turkey Rollups with Veggie Cream Cheese

Prep time: 10 minutes | Cook time: 0 minutes | Serves 2

¼ cup cream cheese, at room temperature
2 tablespoons finely chopped red onion
2 tablespoons finely chopped red bell pepper

1 tablespoon chopped fresh chives
1 teaspoon Dijon mustard
1 garlic clove, minced
¼ teaspoon sea salt
6 slices deli turkey

1. In a small bowl, mix the cream cheese, red onion, bell pepper, chives, mustard, garlic, and salt. 2. Spread the mixture on the turkey slices and roll up.

Per Serving:
calorie: 146 | fat: 1g | protein: 24g | carbs: 8g | sugars: 6g | fiber: 1g | sodium: 572mg

Hummus

Prep time: 5 minutes | Cook time: 5 minutes | Serves 12

One 15-ounce can chickpeas, drained (reserve a little liquid)
3 cloves garlic
Juice of 1 lemon

Juice of 1 lime
1 teaspoon extra-virgin olive oil
1 teaspoon ground cumin

1. In a blender or food processor, combine all the ingredients until smooth, adding chickpea liquid or water if necessary to blend, and create a creamy texture. Refrigerate until ready to serve. Serve with crunchy vegetables, crackers, or pita bread.

Per Serving:
calorie: 56 | fat: 1g | protein: 3g | carbs: 9g | sugars: 2g | fiber: 2g | sodium: 76mg

Lemon Artichokes

Prep time: 5 minutes | Cook time: 5 to 15 minutes | Serves 4

4 artichokes
1 cup water

2 tablespoons lemon juice
1 teaspoon salt

1. Wash and trim artichokes by cutting off the stems flush with the bottoms of the artichokes and by cutting ¾–1 inch off the tops. Stand upright in the bottom of the inner pot of the Instant Pot. 2. Pour water, lemon juice, and salt over artichokes. 3. Secure the lid and make sure the vent is set to sealing. On Manual, set the Instant Pot for 15 minutes for large artichokes, 10 minutes for medium artichokes, or 5 minutes for small artichokes. 4. When cook time is up, perform a quick release by releasing the pressure manually.

Per Serving:
calories: 60 | fat: 0g | protein: 4g | carbs: 13g | sugars: 1g | fiber: 6g | sodium: 397mg

Cucumber Roll-Ups

Prep time: 5 minutes | Cook time: 0 minutes | Serves 2 to 4

2 (6-inch) gluten-free wraps
2 tablespoons cream cheese
1 medium cucumber, cut into

long strips
2 tablespoons fresh mint

1. Place the wraps on your work surface and spread them evenly with the cream cheese. Top with the cucumber and mint. 2. Roll the wraps up from one side to the other, kind of like a burrito. Slice into 1-inch bites or keep whole. 3. Serve. 4. Store any leftovers in an airtight container in the refrigerator for 1 to 2 days.

Per Serving:
calorie: 70 | fat: 1g | protein: 4g | carbs: 12g | sugars: 3g | fiber: 2g | sodium: 183mg

Lemony White Bean Puree

Prep time: 10 minutes | Cook time: 0 minutes | Makes 4 cups

1 (15-ounce) can white beans, drained and rinsed
1 small onion, coarsely chopped
1 garlic clove, minced
Zest and juice of 1 lemon

½ teaspoon herbs de Provence
3 tablespoons extra-virgin olive oil, divided
1 tablespoon chopped fresh parsley

1. Place the beans, onion, garlic, lemon zest and juice, and herbs in a food processor and pulse until smooth. While the machine is running, slowly stream in 2 tablespoons of extra-virgin olive oil. If the mixture is too thick, add water very slowly until you've reached the desired consistency. 2. Transfer the puree to a medium serving bowl. Top with the remaining 1 tablespoon of extra-virgin olive oil and the parsley. 3. Serve with your favorite vegetable or flatbread of choice. Store any leftovers in an airtight container in the refrigerator for up to 4 days.

Per Serving:
calorie: 121 | fat: 5g | protein: 5g | carbs: 15g | sugars: 1g | fiber: 3g | sodium: 4mg

Vegetable Kabobs with Mustard Dip

Prep time: 35 minutes | Cook time: 10 minutes | Serves 9

Dip
⅔ cup plain fat-free yogurt
⅓ cup fat-free sour cream
1 tablespoon finely chopped fresh parsley
1 teaspoon onion powder
1 teaspoon garlic salt
1 tablespoon Dijon mustard
Kabobs

1 medium bell pepper, cut into 6 strips, then cut into thirds
1 medium zucchini, cut diagonally into ½-inch slices
1 package (8 ounces) fresh whole mushrooms
9 large cherry tomatoes
2 tablespoons olive or vegetable oil

1. In small bowl, mix dip ingredients. Cover; refrigerate at least 1 hour. 2. Heat gas or charcoal grill. On 5 (12-inch) metal skewers, thread vegetables so that one kind of vegetable is on the same skewer (use 2 skewers for mushrooms); leave space between each piece. Brush vegetables with oil. 3. Place skewers of bell pepper and zucchini on grill over medium heat. Cover grill; cook 2 minutes. Add skewers of mushrooms and tomatoes. Cover grill; cook 4 to 5 minutes, carefully turning every 2 minutes, until vegetables are tender. Transfer vegetables from skewers to serving plate. Serve with dip.

Per Serving:
calories: 60 | fat: 4g | protein: 2g | carbs: 6g | sugars: 3g | fiber: 1g | sodium: 180mg

Baked Scallops

Prep time: 5 minutes | Cook time: 10 minutes | Serves 4

12 ounces fresh bay or dry sea scallops
1½ teaspoons salt-free pickling spices
½ cup cider vinegar
¼ cup water
1 tablespoon finely chopped

onion
1 red bell pepper, cut into thin strips
1 head butter lettuce, rinsed and dried
⅓ cup sesame seeds, toasted

1. Preheat the oven to 350 degrees. Wash the scallops in cool water, and cut any scallops that are too big in half. 2. Spread the scallops out in a large baking dish (be careful not to overlap them). In a small bowl, combine the spices, cider vinegar, water, onion, and pepper; pour the mixture over the scallops. Season with salt, if desired. 3. Cover the baking dish and bake for 7 minutes. Remove from the oven, and allow the scallops to chill in the refrigerator (leave them in the cooking liquid/vegetable mixture). 4. Just before serving, place the lettuce leaves on individual plates or a platter, and place the scallops and vegetables over the top. Sprinkle with sesame seeds before serving.

Per Serving:
calorie: 159 | fat: 8g | protein: 14g | carbs: 7g | sugars: 2g | fiber: 3g | sodium: 344mg

Roasted Carrot and Chickpea Dip

Prep time: 10 minutes | Cook time: 15 minutes | Makes 4 cups

4 medium carrots, quartered lengthwise
¼ cup plus 2 teaspoons extra-virgin olive oil, divided
Pinch kosher salt
Pinch freshly ground black pepper
1 (15-ounce) can chickpeas, drained and rinsed
1 garlic clove, minced

1 red chile (optional)
Zest and juice of 1 lemon
2 tablespoons tahini
1 tablespoon harissa
½ teaspoon ground cumin
¼ teaspoon ground coriander
Pomegranate arils (seeds) (optional)
Cilantro, chopped (optional)

1. Preheat the oven to 425°F. Line a baking sheet with parchment paper. 2. In a medium bowl, toss the carrots with 2 teaspoons of extra-virgin olive oil, the salt, and the pepper. Spread them in a single layer on the prepared baking sheet and roast until tender, about 15 minutes. Turn the carrots over halfway through. 3. Meanwhile, place the chickpeas, garlic, chile, lemon zest and juice, tahini, harissa, cumin, and coriander in a food processor. Set aside. Add the carrots to the processor when they are cooked. Pulse until the mixture is coarse. Scrape the bowl down, then turn the processor back on while you drizzle the remaining ¼ cup of extra-virgin olive oil through the feed tube of the machine. Adjust the seasonings as desired. If it's too thick, add water to thin. 4. Top with pomegranate seeds and chopped cilantro (if using,) and Serve with cut vegetables. 5. Store any leftovers in an airtight container in the refrigerator for up to 4 days.

Per Serving:
calorie: 141 | fat: 10g | protein: 3g | carbs: 12g | sugars: 3g | fiber: 3g | sodium: 93mg

Creamy Jalapeño Chicken Dip

Prep time: 5 minutes | Cook time: 12 minutes | Serves 10

1 pound boneless chicken breast
8 ounces low-fat cream cheese
3 jalapeños, seeded and sliced
½ cup water

8 ounces reduced-fat shredded cheddar cheese
¾ cup low-fat sour cream

1. Place the chicken, cream cheese, jalapeños, and water in the inner pot of the Instant Pot. 2. Secure the lid so it's locked and turn the vent to sealing. 3. Press Manual and set the Instant Pot for 12 minutes on high pressure. 4. When cooking time is up, turn off Instant Pot, do a quick release of the remaining pressure, then remove lid. 5. Shred the chicken between 2 forks, either in the pot or on a cutting board, then place back in the inner pot. 6. Stir in the shredded cheese and sour cream.

Per Serving:
calories: 238 | fat: 13g | protein: 24g | carbs: 7g | sugars: 5g | fiber: 1g | sodium: 273mg

Smoky Spinach Hummus with Popcorn Chips

Prep time: 10 minutes | Cook time: 0 minutes | Serves 12

1 can (15 ounces) chickpeas (garbanzo beans), drained, liquid reserved	2 teaspoons smoked Spanish paprika
1 cup chopped fresh spinach leaves	1 teaspoon ground cumin
2 tablespoons lemon juice	½ teaspoon salt
2 tablespoons sesame tahini paste (from 16 ounces. jar)	2 tablespoons chopped red bell pepper, if desired
	6 ounces popcorn snack chips

1. In food processor, place chickpeas, ¼ cup of the reserved liquid, spinach, lemon juice, tahini paste, paprika, cumin and salt. Cover; process 30 seconds, using quick on-and-off motions; scrape side. 2. Add additional reserved bean liquid, 1 tablespoon at a time, covering and processing, using quick on-and-off motions, until smooth and desired dipping consistency. Garnish with bell pepper. Serve with popcorn snack chips.

Per Serving:

calories: 140 | fat: 4g | protein: 4g | carbs: 22g | sugars: 0g | fiber: 3g | sodium: 270mg

7-Layer Dip

Prep time: 10 minutes | Cook time: 35 minutes | Serves 6

Cashew Sour Cream	½ teaspoon chili powder
1 cup raw whole cashews, soaked in water to cover for 1 to 2 hours and then drained	¼ teaspoon garlic powder
½ cup avocado oil	½ cup grape or cherry tomatoes, halved
½ cup water	1 avocado, diced
¼ cup fresh lemon juice	¼ cup chopped yellow onion
2 tablespoons nutritional yeast	1 jalapeño chile, sliced
1 teaspoon fine sea salt	2 tablespoons chopped cilantro
Beans	6 ounces baked corn tortilla chips
½ cup dried black beans	1 English cucumber, sliced
2 cups water	2 carrots, sliced
½ teaspoon fine sea salt	6 celery stalks, cut into sticks

1. To make the cashew sour cream: In a blender, combine the cashews, oil, water, lemon juice, nutritional yeast, and salt. Blend on high speed, stopping to scrape down the sides of the container as needed, for about 2 minutes, until very smooth. (The sour cream can be made in advance and stored in an airtight container in the refrigerator for up to 5 days.) 2. To make the beans: Pour 1 cup water into the Instant Pot. In a 1½-quart stainless-steel bowl, combine the beans, the 2 cups water, and salt and stir to dissolve the salt. Place the bowl on a long-handled silicone steam rack, then, holding the handles of the steam rack, lower it into the Instant Pot. (If you don't have the long-handled rack, use the wire metal steam rack and a homemade sling) 3. Secure the lid and set the Pressure Release to Sealing. Select the Bean/Chili, Pressure Cook, or Manual setting

and set the cooking time for 25 minutes at high pressure. (The pot will take about 10 minutes to come up to pressure before the cooking program begins.) 4. When the cooking program ends, let the pressure release naturally for at least 20 minutes, then move the Pressure Release to Venting to release any remaining steam. 5. Place a colander over a bowl. Open the pot and, wearing heat-resistant mitts, lift out the inner pot and drain the beans in the colander. Transfer the liquid captured in the bowl to a measuring cup, and pour the beans into the bowl. Add ¼ cup of the cooking liquid to the beans and, using a potato masher or fork, mash the beans to your desired consistency, adding more cooking liquid as needed. Stir in the chili powder and garlic powder. 6. Using a rubber spatula, spread the black beans in an even layer in a clear-glass serving dish. Spread the cashew sour cream in an even layer on top of the beans. Add layers of the tomatoes, avocado, onion, jalapeño, and cilantro. (At this point, you can cover and refrigerate the assembled dip for up to 1 day.) Serve accompanied with the tortilla chips, cucumber, carrots, and celery on the side.

Per Serving:

calories: 259 | fat: 8g | protein: 8g | carbs: 41g | sugars: 3g | fiber: 8g | sodium: 811mg

Cocoa Coated Almonds

Prep time: 5 minutes | Cook time: 15 minutes | Serves 4

1 cup almonds	2 packets powdered stevia
1 tablespoon cocoa powder	

1. Preheat the oven to 350°F. Line a baking sheet with parchment paper. 2. Spread the almonds in a single layer on the baking sheet. Bake for 5 minutes. 3. While the almonds bake, in a small bowl, mix the cocoa and stevia well. Add the hot almonds to the bowl. Toss to combine. 4. Return the almonds to the baking sheet and bake until fragrant, about 5 minutes more.

Per Serving:

calorie: 143 | fat: 12g | protein: 5g | carbs: 6g | sugars: 1g | fiber: 3g | sodium: 1mg

Garlic Kale Chips

Prep time: 5 minutes | Cook time: 15 minutes | Serves 1

1 (8-ounce) bunch kale, trimmed and cut into 2-inch pieces	½ teaspoon sea salt
	¼ teaspoon garlic powder
1 tablespoon extra-virgin olive oil	Pinch cayenne (optional, to taste)

1. Preheat the oven to 350°F. Line two baking sheets with parchment paper. 2. Wash the kale and pat it completely dry. 3. In a large bowl, toss the kale with the olive oil, sea salt, garlic powder, and cayenne, if using. 4. Spread the kale in a single layer on the prepared baking sheets. 5. Bake until crisp, 12 to 15 minutes, rotating the sheets once.

Per Serving:

calorie: 78 | fat: 5g | protein: 3g | carbs: 7g | sugars: 2g | fiber: 3g | sodium: 416mg

Cucumber Pâté

Prep time: 10 minutes | Cook time: 20 minutes | Serves 12

1 large cucumber, peeled, seeded, and quartered	1 cup low-fat cottage cheese
1 small green bell pepper, seeded and quartered	½ cup plain nonfat Greek yogurt
3 stalks celery, quartered	1 package unflavored gelatin
1 medium onion, quartered	¼ cup boiling water
	¼ cup cold water

1. Spray a 5-cup mold or a 1½-quart mixing bowl with nonstick cooking spray. 2. In a food processor, coarsely chop the cucumber, green pepper, celery, and onion. Remove the vegetables from the food processor and set aside. 3. In a food processor, combine the cottage cheese and yogurt, and blend until smooth. 4. In a medium bowl, dissolve the gelatin in the boiling water; slowly stir in the cold water. Add the chopped vegetables and cottage cheese mixture, and mix thoroughly. 5. Pour the mixture into the prepared mold and refrigerate overnight or until firm. To serve, carefully invert the mold onto a serving plate, and remove the mold. Surround the pâté with assorted crackers, and serve.

Per Serving:

calorie: 57 | fat: 2g | protein: 6g | carbs: 3g | sugars: 2g | fiber: 1g | sodium: 107mg

Blood Sugar–Friendly Nutty Trail Mix

Prep time: 5 minutes | Cook time: 0 minutes | Serves 4

¼ cup (31 g) raw shelled pistachios	¼ cup (38 g) raisins
¼ cup (30 g) raw pecans	¼ cup (45 g) dairy-free dark chocolate chips
¼ cup (43 g) raw almonds	

1. In a medium bowl, combine the pistachios, pecans, almonds, raisins, and chocolate chips. 2. Divide the trail mix into four portions.

Per Serving:

calorie: 234 | fat: 17g | protein: 5g | carbs: 21g | sugars: 15g | fiber: 4g | sodium: 6mg

Gruyere Apple Spread

Prep time: 5 minutes | Cook time: 5 minutes | Serves 20

4 ounces fat-free cream cheese, softened	pepper
½ cup low-fat cottage cheese	½ cup shredded apple (unpeeled)
4 ounces Gruyere cheese	2 tablespoons finely chopped pecans
¼ teaspoon dry mustard	2 teaspoons minced fresh chives
⅛ teaspoon freshly ground black	

1. Place the cheeses in a food processor, and blend until smooth. Add the mustard and pepper, and blend for 30 seconds. 2. Transfer the mixture to a serving bowl, and fold in the apple and pecans. Sprinkle

the dip with chives. 3. Cover, and refrigerate the mixture for 1–2 hours. Serve chilled with crackers, or stuff into celery stalks.

Per Serving:

calorie: 46 | fat: 3g | protein: 4g | carbs: 1g | sugars: 1g | fiber: 0g | sodium: 107mg

Creamy Apple-Cinnamon Quesadilla

Prep time: 15 minutes | Cook time: 10 minutes | Serves 4

1 tablespoon granulated sugar	sugar
½ teaspoon ground cinnamon	2 whole wheat tortillas (8 inch)
¼ cup reduced-fat cream cheese (from 8 ounces container)	½ small apple, cut into ¼-inch slices (½ cup)
1 tablespoon packed brown	Cooking spray

1. In small bowl, mix granulated sugar and ¼ teaspoon of the cinnamon; set aside. In another small bowl, mix cream cheese, brown sugar and remaining ¼ teaspoon cinnamon with spoon. 2. Spread cream cheese mixture over tortillas. Place apple slices on cream cheese mixture on 1 tortilla. Top with remaining tortilla, cheese side down. Spray both sides of quesadilla with cooking spray; sprinkle with cinnamon-sugar mixture. 3. Heat 10-inch nonstick skillet over medium heat. Add quesadilla; cook 2 to 3 minutes or until bottom is brown and crisp. Turn quesadilla; cook 2 to 3 minutes longer or until bottom is brown and crisp. 4. Transfer quesadilla from skillet to cutting board; let stand 2 to 3 minutes. Cut into 8 wedges to serve.

Per Serving:

calories: 110 | fat: 3g | protein: 3g | carbs: 19g | sugars: 9g | fiber: 2g | sodium: 170mg

Sweet Potato Oven Fries with Spicy Sour Cream

Prep time: 10 minutes | Cook time: 35 minutes | Serves 4

1 teaspoon salt-free southwest chipotle seasoning	Olive oil cooking spray
2 large dark-orange sweet potatoes (1 pound), peeled, cut into ½-inch-thick slices	½ cup reduced-fat sour cream
	1 tablespoon sriracha sauce
	1 tablespoon chopped fresh cilantro

1. Heat oven to 425°F. Spray large cookie sheet with cooking spray. Place ¾ teaspoon of the seasoning in 1-gallon resealable food-storage plastic bag; add potatoes. Seal bag; shake until potatoes are evenly coated. Place potatoes in single layer on cookie sheet; spray lightly with cooking spray. Bake 20 minutes or until bottoms are golden brown. Turn potatoes; bake 10 to 15 minutes longer or until tender and bottoms are golden brown. 2. Meanwhile, in small bowl, stir sour cream, sriracha sauce, cilantro and remaining ¼ teaspoon seasoning; refrigerate until ready to serve. 3. Serve fries warm with spicy sour cream.

Per Serving:

calories: 120 | fat: 4g | protein: 2g | carbs: 20g | sugars: 7g | fiber: 3g | sodium: 140mg

Peanut Butter Protein Bites

Prep time: 10 minutes | Cook time: 0 minutes | Makes 16 Balls

½ cup sugar-free peanut butter	cocoa powder
¼ cup (1 scoop) sugar-free peanut butter powder or sugar-free protein powder	2 tablespoons canned coconut milk (or more to adjust consistency)
2 tablespoons unsweetened	

1. In a bowl, mix all ingredients until well combined. 2. Roll into 16 balls. Refrigerate before serving.

Per Serving:

calorie: 59 | fat: 5g | protein: 3g | carbs: 2g | sugars: 1g | fiber: 1g | sodium: 4mg

Ground Turkey Lettuce Cups

Prep time: 5 minutes | Cook time: 30 minutes | Serves 8

3 tablespoons water	1 yellow onion, diced
2 tablespoons soy sauce, tamari, or coconut aminos	2 pounds 93 percent lean ground turkey
3 tablespoons fresh lime juice	½ teaspoon fine sea salt
2 teaspoons Sriracha, plus more for serving	Two 8-ounce cans sliced water chestnuts, drained and chopped
2 tablespoons cold-pressed avocado oil	1 tablespoon cornstarch
2 teaspoons toasted sesame oil	2 hearts romaine lettuce or 2 heads butter lettuce, leaves separated
4 garlic cloves, minced	
1-inch piece fresh ginger, peeled and minced	½ cup roasted cashews (whole or halves and pieces), chopped
2 carrots, diced	1 cup loosely packed fresh cilantro leaves
2 celery stalks, diced	

1. In a small bowl, combine the water, soy sauce, 2 tablespoons of the lime juice, and the Sriracha and mix well. Set aside. 2. Select the Sauté setting on the Instant Pot and heat the avocado oil, sesame oil, garlic, and ginger for 2 minutes, until the garlic is bubbling but not browned. Add the carrots, celery, and onion and sauté for about 3 minutes, until the onion begins to soften. 3. Add the turkey and salt and sauté, using a wooden spoon or spatula to break up the meat as it cooks, for about 5 minutes, until cooked through and no streaks of pink remain. Add the water chestnuts and soy sauce mixture and stir to combine, working quickly so not too much steam escapes. 4. Secure the lid and set the Pressure Release to Sealing. Press the Cancel button to reset the cooking program, then select the Pressure Cook or Manual setting and set the cooking time for 5 minutes at high pressure. (The pot will take about 10 minutes to come up to pressure before the cooking program begins.) 5. When the cooking program ends, perform a quick pressure release by moving the Pressure Release to Venting, or let the pressure release naturally. Open the pot. 6. In a small bowl, stir together the remaining 1 tablespoon lime juice and the cornstarch, add the mixture to the pot, and stir to combine. Press the Cancel button to reset the cooking program, then select the Sauté setting. Let the mixture come to a boil and thicken, stirring often, for about 2 minutes, then press the Cancel button to turn off the pot. 7. Spoon the turkey mixture onto the lettuce leaves and sprinkle the cashews and cilantro on top. Serve right away, with additional Sriracha at the table.

Per Serving:

calories: 127 | fat: 7g | protein: 6g | carbs: 10g | sugars: 2g | fiber: 3g | sodium: 392mg

No-Bake Coconut and Cashew Energy Bars

Prep time: 5 minutes | Cook time: 0 minutes | Makes 12 energy bars

1 cup (110 g) raw cashews	butter of choice
1 cup (80 g) unsweetened shredded coconut	2 tablespoons (30 ml) pure maple syrup
½ cup (120 g) unsweetened nut	

1. Line an 8 x 8–inch (20 x 20–cm) baking pan with parchment paper. 2. In a large food processor, combine the cashews and coconut. Pulse them for 15 to 20 seconds to form a powder. 3. Add the nut butter and maple syrup and process until a doughy paste is formed, scraping down the sides if needed. 4. Spread the dough into the prepared baking pan. Cover the dough with another sheet of parchment paper and press it flat. 5. Freeze the dough for 1 hour. Cut the dough into bars.

Per Serving:

calorie: 169 | fat: 14g | protein: 4g | carbs: 10g | sugars: 3g | fiber: 2g | sodium: 6mg

Broiled Shrimp with Garlic

Prep time: 5 minutes | Cook time: 10 minutes | Serves 12

2 pounds large shrimp, unshelled	2 teaspoons freshly ground black pepper
⅓ cup extra-virgin olive oil	1 large lemon, sliced
1 tablespoon lemon juice	4 tablespoons chopped fresh parsley
¼ cup chopped scallions	
1 tablespoon chopped garlic	

1. Set the oven to broil. Shell the uncooked shrimp, but do not remove the tails. With a small knife, split the shrimp down the back, and remove the vein. Wash the shrimp with cool water, and pat dry with paper towels. 2. In a medium skillet, over medium heat, heat the olive oil. Add the lemon juice, scallions, garlic, and pepper. Heat the mixture for 3 minutes. Set aside. 3. In a baking dish, arrange the shrimp and pour the olive oil mixture over the shrimp. Broil the shrimp 4–5 inches from the heat for 2 minutes per side, just until the shrimp turns bright pink. Transfer the shrimp to a platter and garnish with lemon slices and parsley. Pour the juices from the pan over the shrimp.

Per Serving:

calorie: 92 | fat: 3g | protein: 15g | carbs: 1g | sugars: 0g | fiber: 0g | sodium: 142mg

Lemon Cream Fruit Dip

Prep time: 5 minutes | Cook time: 0 minutes | Serves 4

1 cup (200 g) plain nonfat Greek yogurt
¼ cup (28 g) coconut flour 1 tablespoon (15 ml) pure maple syrup
½ teaspoon pure vanilla extract

½ teaspoon pure almond extract
Zest of 1 medium lemon
Juice of ½ medium lemon

1. In a medium bowl, whisk together the yogurt, coconut flour, maple syrup, vanilla, almond extract, lemon zest, and lemon juice. Serve the dip with fruit or crackers.

Per Serving:

calorie: 80 | fat: 1g | protein: 7g | carbs: 10g | sugars: 6g | fiber: 3g | sodium: 37mg

Ginger and Mint Dip with Fruit

Prep time: 20 minutes | Cook time: 0 minutes | Serves 6

Dip
1¼ cups plain fat-free yogurt
¼ cup packed brown sugar
2 teaspoons chopped fresh mint leaves
2 teaspoons grated gingerroot

½ teaspoon grated lemon peel
Fruit Skewers
12 bamboo skewers (6 inch)
1 cup fresh raspberries
2 cups melon cubes (cantaloupe and/or honeydew)

1. In small bowl, mix dip ingredients with whisk until smooth. Cover; refrigerate at least 15 minutes to blend flavors. 2. On each skewer, alternately thread 3 raspberries and 2 melon cubes. Serve with dip.

Per Serving:

calories: 100 | fat: 0g | protein: 3g | carbs: 20g | sugars: 17g | fiber: 2g | sodium: 50mg

Almond Milk Nut Butter Mocha Smoothie

Prep time: 5 minutes | Cook time: 0 minutes | Serves 1

1 cup almond milk
2 tablespoons almond butter
1 tablespoon cocoa powder
1 teaspoon espresso powder (or to taste)

1 to 2 (1-gram) packets stevia (or to taste)
¼ teaspoon almond extract
½ cup crushed ice

1. In a blender, combine all of the ingredients and blend on high until smooth.

Per Serving:

calorie: 249 | fat: 21g | protein: 9g | carbs: 12g | sugars: 2g | fiber: 6g | sodium: 174mg

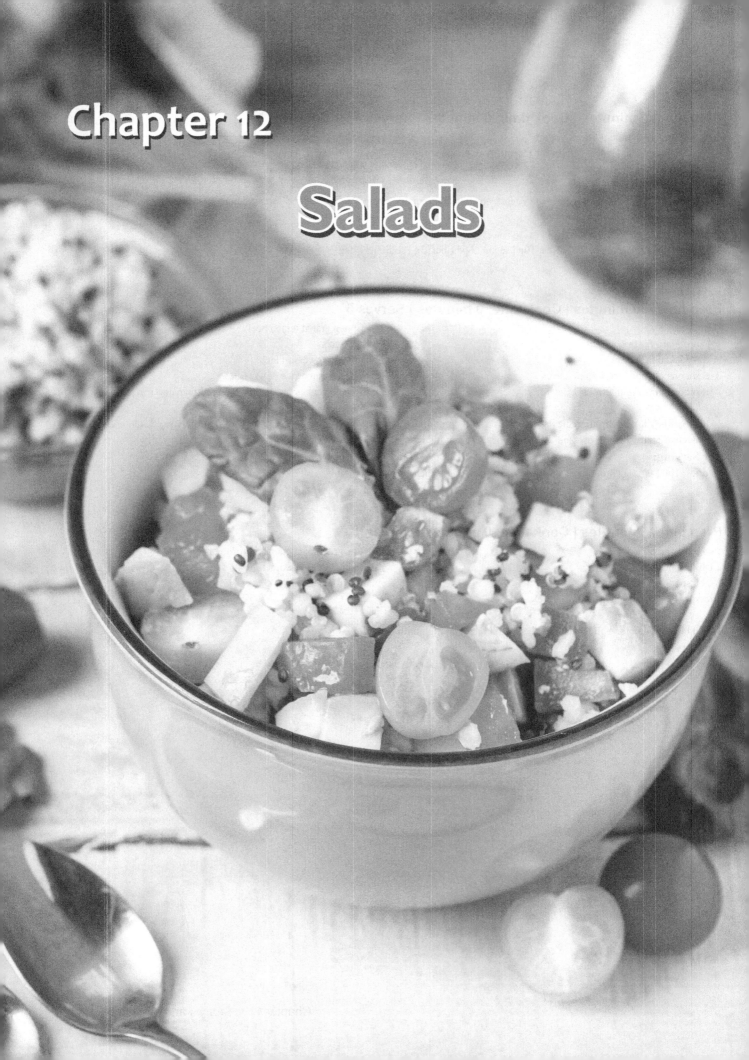

Chapter 12

Salads

Raw Corn Salad with Black-Eyed Peas

Prep time: 15 minutes | Cook time: 0 minutes | Serves 8

2 ears fresh corn, kernels cut off	vinegar
2 cups cooked black-eyed peas	2 tablespoons extra-virgin olive oil
1 green bell pepper, chopped	
½ red onion, chopped	1 garlic clove, minced
2 celery stalks, finely chopped	¼ teaspoon smoked paprika
½ pint cherry tomatoes, halved	¼ teaspoon ground cumin
3 tablespoons white balsamic	¼ teaspoon red pepper flakes

1. In a large salad bowl, combine the corn, black-eyed peas, bell pepper, onion, celery, and tomatoes. 2. In a small bowl, to make the dressing, whisk the vinegar, olive oil, garlic, paprika, cumin, and red pepper flakes together. 3. Pour the dressing over the salad, and toss gently to coat. Serve and enjoy.

Per Serving:

calorie: 127 | fat: 4g | protein: 5g | carbs: 19g | sugars: 5g | fiber: 5g | sodium: 16mg

Carrot and Cashew Chicken Salad

Prep time: 20 minutes | Cook time: 25 minutes | Serves 2

Extra-virgin olive oil cooking spray	1 (6-ounce) boneless skinless chicken breast, thinly sliced across the grain
1 cup carrots rounds	
1 red bell pepper, thinly sliced	2 tablespoons chopped scallions
1½ teaspoons granulated stevia	1 tablespoon apple cider vinegar
1 tablespoon extra-virgin olive oil, divided	1 cup sugar snap peas
	4 cups baby spinach
¼ teaspoon salt, divided	4 tablespoons chopped cashews, divided
⅜ teaspoon freshly ground black pepper, divided	

1. Preheat the oven to 425°F. 2. Coat an 8-by-8-inch baking pan and a rimmed baking sheet with cooking spray. 3. In the prepared baking pan, add the carrots and red bell pepper. Sprinkle with the stevia, 1 teaspoon of olive oil, ⅛ teaspoon of salt, and ⅛ teaspoon of pepper. Toss to coat. 4. Place the pan in the preheated oven. Roast for about 25 minutes, stirring several times, or until tender. 5. About 5 minutes before the vegetables are done, place the sliced chicken in a medium bowl and drizzle with 1 teaspoon of olive oil. Sprinkle with the scallions. Season with the remaining ⅛ teaspoon of salt and ⅛ teaspoon of pepper. Toss to mix. Arrange in a single layer on the prepared baking sheet. 6. Place the sheet in the preheated oven. Roast for 5 to 7 minutes, turning once, or until cooked through. 7. Remove the pan with the vegetables and the baking sheet from the oven. Cool for about 3 minutes. 8. In a large salad bowl, mix together the apple cider vinegar, the remaining 1 teaspoon of olive oil, the sugar snap peas, and remaining ⅛ teaspoon of pepper. Let stand 5 minutes to blend the flavors. 9. To finish, add the spinach to the bowl with the dressing and peas. Toss to mix well. 10. Evenly divide between 2 serving plates. Top each with half of the roasted carrots, half of the roasted red bell peppers, and half of the cooked chicken. 11. Sprinkle each with about 2 tablespoons of cashews. Serve warm.

Per Serving:

calorie: 335 | fat: 17g | protein: 26g | carbs: 21g | sugars: 8g | fiber: 6g | sodium: 422mg

Herbed Tomato Salad

Prep time: 7 minutes | Cook time: 0 minutes | Serves 2 to 4

1 pint cherry tomatoes, halved	1 teaspoon sumac (optional)
1 bunch fresh parsley, leaves only (stems discarded)	2 tablespoons extra-virgin olive oil
1 cup cilantro, leaves only (stems discarded)	Kosher salt
¼ cup fresh dill	Freshly ground black pepper

1. In a medium bowl, carefully toss together the tomatoes, parsley, cilantro, dill, sumac (if using), extra-virgin olive oil, and salt and pepper to taste. 2. Store any leftovers in an airtight container in the refrigerator for up to 3 days, but the salad is best consumed on the day it is dressed.

Per Serving:

calorie: 113 | fat: 10g | protein: 2g | carbs: 7g | sugars: 3g | fiber: 3g | sodium: 30mg

Mediterranean Pasta Salad with Goat Cheese

Prep time: 25 minutes | Cook time: 0 minutes | Serves 4

½ cup (75 g) grape tomatoes, sliced in half lengthwise	sea salt
	½ teaspoon black pepper
1 medium red bell pepper, coarsely chopped	1 tablespoon (3 g) dried oregano
½ medium red onion, sliced into thin strips	½ teaspoon garlic powder
	4 ounces (113 g) crumbled goat cheese
1 medium zucchini, coarsely chopped	½ cup (50 g) shaved Parmesan cheese
1 cup (175 g) broccoli florets	8 ounces (227 g) lentil or chickpea penne pasta, cooked, rinsed, and drained
½ cup (110 g) oil-packed artichoke hearts, drained	
¼ cup (60 ml) olive oil	

1. In a large bowl, combine the tomatoes, bell pepper, onion, zucchini, broccoli, artichoke hearts, oil, sea salt, black pepper, oregano, garlic powder, goat cheese, and Parmesan cheese. Gently mix everything together to combine and coat all of the ingredients with the oil. 2. Add the pasta to the bowl and stir to combine. 3. Let the pasta salad rest for 1 to 2 hours in the refrigerator to marinate it, or serve the pasta salad immediately if desired.

Per Serving:

calorie: 477 | fat: 24g | protein: 23g | carbs: 41g | sugars: 6g | fiber: 6g | sodium: 706mg

Cheeseburger Wedge Salad

Prep time: 15 minutes | Cook time: 10 minutes | Serves 4

salad
1 pound (454 g) lean ground beef
2 medium heads romaine lettuce, rinsed, dried, and sliced in half lengthwise
½ cup (60 g) shredded Cheddar cheese
½ cup (80 g) coarsely chopped tomatoes
⅓ cup (50 g) finely chopped red onion

1 small dill pickle, finely chopped (optional)
dressing
2 ounces (57 g) no-salt-added tomato paste
2 tablespoons (30 ml) apple cider vinegar
2 tablespoons (30 ml) water
1 tablespoon (15 ml) honey
¼ teaspoon sea salt
½ teaspoon onion powder
¼ teaspoon garlic powder

1. To make the salad, heat a large skillet over medium-high heat. Once the skillet is hot, add the beef and cook it for 9 to 10 minutes, until it is brown and cooked though. 2. Meanwhile, place a ½ head of romaine lettuce on each of four plates. Divide the beef evenly on top of each of the romaine halves. Then top each with the Cheddar cheese, tomatoes, onion, and pickle (if using). 3. To make the dressing, combine the tomato paste, vinegar, water, honey, sea salt, onion powder, and garlic powder in a small mason jar, secure the lid on top, and shake the jar thoroughly until everything is combined. Drizzle the dressing evenly over each salad and serve.

Per Serving:

calorie: 320 | fat: 14g | protein: 32g | carbs: 19g | sugars: 11g | fiber: 8g | sodium: 341mg

Crunchy Pecan Tuna Salad

Prep time: 20 minutes | Cook time: 0 minutes | Serves 1

½ medium apple, finely chopped
2 medium ribs celery, finely chopped
¼ large red onion, finely chopped
2 tablespoons (16 g) coarsely chopped pecans
¼ cup (46 g) canned navy beans, drained, rinsed, and mashed

2 ounces (57 g) canned tuna packed in water, drained and rinsed
1 tablespoon (14 g) mayonnaise (see Tip)
½ tablespoon (8 g) Dijon mustard
1 tablespoon (15 ml) fresh lemon juice
Black pepper, as needed

1. In a large bowl, combine the apple, celery, onion, pecans, beans, and tuna. 2. In a small bowl, mix together the mayonnaise, mustard, lemon juice, and black pepper. Add the mayonnaise mixture to the tuna mixture and stir until the tuna salad is evenly combined. 3. Serve the tuna salad immediately, or refrigerate the tuna salad for 2 to 3 hours or overnight to chill it and allow the flavors to meld.

Per Serving:

calorie: 197 | fat: 11g | protein: 11g | carbs: 16g | sugars: 7g | fiber: 5g | sodium: 179mg

Strawberry-Spinach Salad

Prep time: 15 minutes | Cook time: 0 minutes | Serves 4

½ cup extra-virgin olive oil
¼ cup balsamic vinegar
1 tablespoon Worcestershire sauce
1 (10-ounce) package baby spinach
1 medium red onion, quartered

and sliced
1 cup strawberries, sliced
1 (6-ounce) container feta cheese, crumbled
4 tablespoons bacon bits, divided
1 cup slivered almonds, divided

1. In a large bowl, whisk together the olive oil, balsamic vinegar, and Worcestershire sauce. 2. Add the spinach, onion, strawberries, and feta cheese and mix until all the ingredients are coated. 3. Portion into 4 servings and top each with 1 tablespoon of bacon bits and ¼ cup of slivered almonds.

Per Serving:

calorie: 417 | fat: 29g | protein: 24g | carbs: 19g | sugars: 7g | fiber: 7g | sodium: 542mg

Strawberry-Blueberry-Orange Salad

Prep time: 15 minutes | Cook time: 0 minutes | Serves 8

¼ cup fat-free or reduced-fat mayonnaise
3 tablespoons sugar
1 tablespoon white vinegar
2 teaspoons poppy seed

2 cups fresh strawberry halves
2 cups fresh blueberries
1 orange, peeled, chopped
Sliced almonds, if desired

1. In small bowl, mix mayonnaise, sugar, vinegar and poppy seed with whisk until well blended. 2. In medium bowl, mix strawberries, blueberries and orange. Just before serving, pour dressing over fruit; toss. Sprinkle with almonds.

Per Serving:

calorie: 70 | fat: 1g | protein: 0g | carbs: 16g | sugars: 12g | fiber: 2g | sodium: 60mg

Nutty Deconstructed Salad

Prep time: 10 minutes | Cook time: 0 minutes | Serves 1

6 ounces (170 g) grilled or baked chicken, sliced or cubed to the desired size
½ cup (75 g) red seedless grapes
¼ cup (32 g) crumbled feta

cheese
¼ cup (30 g) raw walnuts
2 tablespoons (10 g) raw pumpkin seeds
1 small apple, thinly sliced

1. In a salad bowl, combine the chicken, grapes, feta cheese, walnuts, pumpkin seeds, and apple. Toss to combine the ingredients and serve.

Per Serving:

calorie: 613 | fat: 33g | protein: 42g | carbs: 42g | sugars: 30g | fiber: 6g | sodium: 501mg

Rotisserie Chicken and Avocado Salad

Prep time: 15 minutes | Cook time: 0 minutes | Serves 4

½ cup plain Greek yogurt
1 tablespoon freshly squeezed lime juice
4 teaspoons chopped fresh cilantro
2 ripe avocados, peeled, pitted, and cubed

1 cup shredded rotisserie chicken meat
½ medium red onion, chopped
1 large tomato, diced
4 cups mixed leafy greens, divided

1. In a large bowl, stir together the Greek yogurt, lime juice, and cilantro to make a dressing. 2. Add the avocado, chicken, onion, and tomato and mix gently into the dressing. 3. Divide 1 cup of the greens into 4 bowls and top with the chicken salad.

Per Serving:

calorie: 269 | fat: 18g | protein: 14g | carbs: 16g | sugars: 5g | fiber: 9g | sodium: 93mg

Mediterranean Chicken Salad

Prep time: 5 minutes | Cook time: 0 minutes | Serves 3

8 ounces boneless, skinless, cooked chicken breast
2 tablespoons extra-virgin olive oil
2 tablespoons balsamic vinegar
¼ teaspoon dried basil
2 small garlic cloves, minced
¼ teaspoon freshly ground black

pepper
1 cup cooked green beans, cut into 2-inch pieces
1 cup cooked artichokes
¼ cup pine nuts, toasted
¼ cup sliced black olives
3 cherry tomatoes, halved
Tomato wedges (optional)

1. Cut the cooked chicken into bite-sized chunks, and set aside. 2. In a medium bowl, whisk together the oil, vinegar, basil, garlic, and pepper. Add the chicken, and toss with the dressing. 3. Add the green beans, artichokes, pine nuts, olives, and cherry tomatoes; toss well. Chill in the refrigerator for several hours. Garnish the salad with tomato wedges, and serve.

Per Serving:

calorie: 307 | fat: 19g | protein: 21g | carbs: 14g | sugars: 4g | fiber: 7g | sodium: 73mg

Three-Bean Salad with Black Bean Crumbles

Prep time: 15 minutes | Cook time: 0 minutes | Serves 4

½ cup bottled Italian dressing
2 cups frozen black bean crumbles, microwaved per package instructions
1 cup cherry tomatoes, halved
1 (16-ounce) can or jar three-

bean salad mix, drained
1 medium onion, quartered and thinly sliced
4 cups romaine salad greens
1 cup shredded reduced-fat cheddar cheese, divided

1. Pour the Italian dressing into a large bowl. Add the black bean crumbles, cherry tomatoes, three-bean salad, and onion and mix until everything is well coated. 2. Divide the greens into 4 bowls and top each with the bean mixture. 3. Sprinkle ¼ cup of shredded cheddar cheese on each portion.

Per Serving:

calorie: 357 | fat: 10g | protein: 22g | carbs: 48g | sugars: 6g | fiber: 9g | sodium: 478mg

Apple-Bulgur Salad

Prep time: 10 minutes | Cook time: 15 minutes | Serves 2

2 cups water
1 cup bulgur
1 teaspoon dried thyme
2 tablespoons extra-virgin olive oil
2 teaspoons cider vinegar

Kosher salt
Freshly ground black pepper
6 kale leaves, shredded
1 small apple, cored and diced
3 tablespoons sliced, toasted almonds

1. In a large saucepan, bring the water to a boil over high heat and remove it from the heat. Add the bulgur and thyme, cover, and allow the grain to rest for 7 to 15 minutes or until cooked through. 2. Meanwhile, in a large bowl, whisk together the extra-virgin olive oil and cider vinegar with a pinch of salt and pepper. Add the cooked bulgur, kale, apple, and almonds to the dressing and toss to combine. Adjust the seasonings as desired. 3. Store any leftovers in an airtight container in the refrigerator for 3 to 5 days.

Per Serving:

calorie: 496 | fat: 22g | protein: 13g | carbs: 69g | sugars: 9g | fiber: 13g | sodium: 33mg

Wild Rice Salad

Prep time: 5 minutes | Cook time: 45 minutes | Serves 6

1 cup raw wild rice (rinsed)
4 cups cold water
1 cup mandarin oranges, packed in their own juice (drain and reserve 2 tablespoons of liquid)
½ cup chopped celery

¼ cup minced red bell pepper
1 shallot, minced
1 teaspoon minced thyme
2 tablespoons raspberry vinegar
1 tablespoon extra-virgin olive oil

1. Place the rinsed, raw rice and the water in a saucepan. Bring to a boil, lower the heat, cover the pan, and cook for 45–50 minutes until the rice has absorbed the water. Set the rice aside to cool. 2. In a large bowl, combine the mandarin oranges, celery, red pepper, and shallot. 3. In a small bowl, combine the reserved juice, thyme, vinegar, and oil. 4. Add the rice to the mandarin oranges and vegetables. Pour the dressing over the salad, toss, and serve.

Per Serving:

calorie: 134 | fat: 3g | protein: 4g | carbs: 24g | sugars: 4g | fiber: 3g | sodium: 12mg

Herbed Spring Peas

Prep time: 10 minutes | Cook time: 15 minutes | Serves 6

1 tablespoon unsalted non-hydrogenated plant-based butter	vegetable broth
½ Vidalia onion, thinly sliced	3 cups fresh shelled peas
1 cup store-bought low-sodium	1 tablespoon minced fresh tarragon

1. In a skillet, melt the butter over medium heat. 2. Add the onion and sauté for 2 to 3 minutes, or until the onion is translucent. 3. Add the broth, and reduce the heat to low. 4. Add the peas and tarragon, cover, and cook for 7 to 10 minutes, or until the peas soften. 5. Serve.

Per Serving:

calorie: 43 | fat: 2g | protein: 2g | carbs: 6g | sugars: 3g | fiber: 2g | sodium: 159mg

Chicken Salad with Apricots

Prep time: 10 minutes | Cook time: 0 minutes | Makes 4 cups

1 cup plain Greek yogurt	12 ounces cooked rotisserie chicken, shredded
2 tablespoons minced shallots	
1 teaspoon ground coriander	2 cups chopped celery with the leaves
1 teaspoon Dijon mustard (optional)	¼ cup slivered almonds, toasted
1 tablespoon freshly squeezed lemon juice	¼ cup thinly sliced dried apricots
¼ teaspoon cayenne pepper	1 bunch fresh parsley, chopped

1. In a medium bowl, mix together the Greek yogurt, shallots, coriander, mustard (if using), lemon juice, and cayenne until well combined. 2. Add the chicken, celery, almonds, apricots, and parsley. 3. Serve on your food of choice (lettuce, crackers, jicama slices, radish slices—you name it). 4. Store any leftovers in an airtight container in the refrigerator for up to 3 days.

Per Serving:

calorie: 232 | fat: 7g | protein: 31g | carbs: 11g | sugars: 7g | fiber: 3g | sodium: 152mg

Savory Skillet Corn Bread

Prep time: 15 minutes | Cook time: 20 minutes | Serves 8

Nonstick cooking spray	1 large zucchini, grated
1 cup whole-wheat all-purpose flour	1 cup reduced-fat Cheddar cheese, grated
1 cup yellow cornmeal	¼ bunch chives, finely chopped
1¾ teaspoons baking powder	1 cup buttermilk
¾ teaspoon baking soda	2 large eggs
½ teaspoon salt	3 tablespoons canola oil

1. Preheat the oven to 420°F. Lightly spray a cast iron skillet with cooking spray. 2. In a medium bowl, whisk the flour, cornmeal, baking powder, baking soda, and salt together. 3. In a large bowl, gently whisk the zucchini, cheese, chives, buttermilk, eggs, and oil

together. 4. Add the dry ingredients to the wet ingredients, and stir until just combined, taking care not to overmix, and pour into the prepared skillet. 5. Transfer the skillet to the oven, and bake for 20 minutes, or until a knife inserted into the center comes out clean. Remove from the oven, and let sit for 10 minutes before serving.

Per Serving:

calorie: 239 | fat: 8g | protein: 10g | carbs: 31g | sugars: 3g | fiber: 2g | sodium: 470mg

Sofrito Steak Salad

Prep time: 10 minutes | Cook time: 15 minutes | Serves 4

4 ounces recaíto cooking base	2 cups diced tomato
2 (4-ounce) flank steaks	2 avocados, diced
8 cups fresh spinach, loosely packed	2 cups diced cucumber
	⅓ cup crumbled feta
½ cup sliced red onion	

1. Heat a large skillet over medium-low heat. When hot, pour in the recaíto cooking base, add the steaks, and cover. Cook for 8 to 12 minutes. 2. Meanwhile, divide the spinach into four portions. Top each portion with one-quarter of the onion, tomato, avocados, and cucumber. 3. Remove the steak from the skillet, and let it rest for about 2 minutes before slicing. Place one-quarter of the steak and feta on top of each portion.

Per Serving:

calorie: 314 | fat: 21g | protein: 19g | carbs: 17g | sugars: 5g | fiber: 10g | sodium: 204mg

Sweet Beet Grain Bowl

Prep time: 10 minutes | Cook time: 20 minutes | Serves 2

3 cups water	pepper
1 cup farro, rinsed	4 small cooked beets, sliced
2 tablespoons extra-virgin olive oil	1 pear, cored and diced
	6 cups mixed greens
1 tablespoon honey	⅓ cup pumpkin seeds, roasted
3 tablespoons cider vinegar	¼ cup ricotta cheese
Pinch freshly ground black	

1. In a medium saucepan, stir together the water and farro over high heat and bring to a boil. Reduce the heat to medium and simmer until the farro is tender, 15 to 20 minutes. Drain and rinse the farro under cold running water until cool. Set aside. 2. Meanwhile, in a small bowl, whisk together the extra-virgin olive oil, honey, and vinegar. Season with black pepper. 3. Evenly divide the farro between two bowls. Top each with the beets, pear, greens, pumpkin seeds, and ricotta. Drizzle the bowls with the dressing before serving and adjust the seasonings as desired.

Per Serving:

calorie: 750 | fat: 28g | protein: 21g | carbs: 104g | sugars: 18g | fiber: 12g | sodium: 174mg

Kidney Bean Salad

Prep time: 10 minutes | Cook time: 0 minutes | Serves 4

3 cups diced cucumber	1 cup cooked corn
1 (15-ounce) can low-sodium dark red kidney beans, drained and rinsed	¾ cup sliced red onion
	1 tablespoon extra-virgin olive oil
2 avocados, diced	1 tablespoon apple cider vinegar
1½ cups diced tomatoes	

1. In a large bowl, combine the cucumber, kidney beans, avocados, tomatoes, corn, onion, olive oil, and vinegar.

Per Serving:

calorie: 394 | fat: 20g | protein: 13g | carbs: 47g | sugars: 10g | fiber: 16g | sodium: 261mg

Garden-Fresh Greek Salad

Prep time: 20 minutes | Cook time: 0 minutes | Serves 6

Dressing	1 bag (10 ounces) ready-to-eat romaine lettuce
3 tablespoons fresh lemon juice	
1 tablespoon chopped fresh or 1 teaspoon dried oregano leaves	¾ cup chopped seeded peeled cucumber
½ teaspoon salt	½ cup sliced red onion
½ teaspoon sugar	¼ cup sliced kalamata olives
½ teaspoon Dijon mustard	2 medium tomatoes, seeded, chopped (1½ cups)
¼ teaspoon pepper	
1 clove garlic, finely chopped	¼ cup reduced-fat feta cheese
Salad	

1. In small bowl, beat all dressing ingredients with whisk. 2. In large bowl, toss all salad ingredients except cheese. Stir in dressing until salad is well coated. Sprinkle with cheese.

Per Serving:

calorie: 45 | fat: 2g | protein: 3g | carbs: 6g | sugars: 3g | fiber: 2g | sodium: 340mg

Zucchini, Carrot, and Fennel Salad

Prep time: 10 minutes | Cook time: 8 minutes | Serves ½ cup

2 medium carrots, peeled and julienned	½ teaspoon dried thyme
1 medium zucchini, julienned	1 tablespoon finely minced parsley
½ medium fennel bulb, core removed and julienned	½ teaspoon salt
1 tablespoon fresh orange juice	¼ teaspoon freshly ground black pepper
2 tablespoons Dijon mustard	
3 tablespoons extra-virgin olive oil	¼ cup chopped walnuts
	1 medium head romaine lettuce, washed and leaves separated
1 teaspoon white wine vinegar	

1. Place the carrots, zucchini, and fennel in a medium bowl; set aside. 2. In a medium bowl, combine the orange juice, mustard, olive oil, vinegar, thyme, parsley, salt, and pepper; mix well. 3. Pour the dressing over the vegetables and toss. Add the walnuts, and mix again. Refrigerate until ready to serve. 4. To serve, line a bowl or plates with lettuce leaves, and spoon ½ cup of salad on top.

Per Serving:

calorie: 201 | fat: 16g | protein: 5g | carbs: 14g | sugars: 6g | fiber: 6g | sodium: 285mg

Crab and Rice Salad

Prep time: 10 minutes | Cook time: 50 minutes | Serves 4

1 cup uncooked brown rice	parsley
5 ounces cooked fresh crabmeat, flaked	2 tablespoons minced red onion
	½ cup plain fat-free yogurt
1 large tomato, diced	1½ tablespoons lemon juice
One 1.8-ounce can sliced water chestnuts, drained	¼ teaspoon freshly ground black pepper
¼ cup chopped green bell pepper	1 head butter lettuce, cored and quartered
3 tablespoons chopped fresh	1 large tomato, cut into wedges

1. In a medium saucepan, boil 2½ cups of water. Slowly add the brown rice. Cover, and reduce the heat to low. Cook the rice for 45–50 minutes until tender. Do not continually stir the rice (this will cause it to become gummy). Just check it occasionally. 2. In a large salad bowl, combine all the ingredients except the lettuce and tomato wedges. Just before serving, line 4 plates with the lettuce, and spoon the salad on top of the lettuce. Garnish with the tomato wedges.

Per Serving:

calorie: 253 | fat: 2g | protein: 15g | carbs: 45g | sugars: 6g | fiber: 4g | sodium: 189mg

Three Bean and Basil Salad

Prep time: 10 minutes | Cook time: 0 minutes | Serves 8

1 (15 ounces) can low-sodium chickpeas, drained and rinsed	white and green parts
	¼ cup finely chopped fresh basil
1 (15 ounces) can low-sodium kidney beans, drained and rinsed	3 garlic cloves, minced
	2 tablespoons extra-virgin olive oil
1 (15 ounces) can low-sodium white beans, drained and rinsed	1 tablespoon red wine vinegar
1 red bell pepper, seeded and finely chopped	1 teaspoon Dijon mustard
	¼ teaspoon freshly ground black pepper
¼ cup chopped scallions, both	

1. In a large mixing bowl, combine the chickpeas, kidney beans, white beans, bell pepper, scallions, basil, and garlic. Toss gently to combine. 2. In a small bowl, combine the olive oil, vinegar, mustard, and pepper. Toss with the salad. 3. Cover and refrigerate for an hour before serving, to allow the flavors to mix.

Per Serving:

Calorie: 193 | fat: 5g | protein: 10g | carbs: 29g | sugars: 3g | fiber: 8g | sodium: 246mg

Couscous Salad

Prep time: 10 minutes | Cook time: 6 minutes | Serves ½ cup

1 cup whole-wheat couscous	oil
2 cups boiling water	4 tablespoons rice vinegar
¼ cup finely chopped red or yellow bell pepper	2 garlic cloves, minced
¼ cup chopped carrots	3 tablespoons finely minced scallions
¼ cup finely chopped celery	¼ cup slivered almonds
2 tablespoons minced Italian parsley	¼ teaspoon freshly ground black pepper
1 tablespoon extra-virgin olive	

1. Place dry couscous in a heat-proof bowl. Pour boiling water over it, and let sit for 5–10 minutes until all the water is absorbed. 2. In a large bowl, combine the couscous, bell pepper, carrots, celery, and parsley together. 3. In a blender or food processor, combine the olive oil, vinegar, garlic, and scallions, and process for 1 minute. Pour over the couscous and vegetables, toss well, garnish with almonds, and season with the pepper. Serve.

Per Serving:

calorie: 373 | fat: 15g | protein: 12g | carbs: 51g | sugars: 3g | fiber: 10g | sodium: 34mg

Triple-Berry and Jicama Spinach Salad

Prep time: 30 minutes | Cook time: 0 minutes | Serves 6

Dressing	¼ teaspoon salt
¼ cup fresh raspberries	1 small clove garlic, crushed
3 tablespoons hot pepper jelly	Salad
2 tablespoons canola oil	1 bag (6 ounces) fresh baby spinach leaves
2 tablespoons raspberry vinegar or red wine vinegar	1 cup bite-size strips (1x¼x¼ inch) peeled jicama
2 medium jalapeño chiles, seeded, finely chopped (2 tablespoons)	1 cup fresh blackberries
	1 cup fresh raspberries
2 teaspoons finely chopped shallot	1 cup sliced fresh strawberries

1. In small food processor or blender, combine all dressing ingredients; process until smooth. 2. In large bowl, toss spinach and ¼ cup of the dressing. On 6 serving plates, arrange salad. To serve, top each salad with jicama, blackberries, raspberries, strawberries and drizzle with scant 1 tablespoon of remaining dressing.

Per Serving:

calorie: 120 | fat: 5g | protein: 2g | carbs: 18g | sugars: 9g | fiber: 5g | sodium: 125mg

Sunflower-Tuna-Cauliflower Salad

Prep time: 30 minutes | Cook time: 0 minutes | Serves 2

1 (5-ounce) can tuna packed in water, drained	1 scallion, chopped
½ cup plain nonfat Greek yogurt	¼ cup sunflower seeds
1 teaspoon freshly squeezed lemon juice	2 cups fresh chopped cauliflower florets
1 teaspoon dried dill	4 cups mixed salad greens, divided

1. In a medium bowl, mix together the tuna, yogurt, lemon juice, dill, scallion, and sunflower seeds. 2. Add the cauliflower. Toss gently to coat. 3. Cover and refrigerate for at least 2 hours before serving, stirring occasionally. 4. Serve half of the tuna mixture atop 2 cups of salad greens.

Per Serving:

calorie: 251 | fat: 11g | protein: 24g | carbs: 18g | sugars: 8g | fiber: 7g | sodium: 288mg

Broccoli "Tabouli"

Prep time: 15 minutes | Cook time: 0 minutes | Serves 2

1 broccoli head, trimmed into florets (about 2 cups)	¼ cup chopped red onion
	¼ cup freshly squeezed lemon juice
1 large jicama, peeled	
1 cup chickpeas, drained and rinsed	2 tablespoons sunflower seeds
	1 tablespoon extra-virgin olive oil
2 plum tomatoes, diced	
1 medium cucumber, peeled, seeded, and diced	Salt, to season
	Freshly ground black pepper, to season
½ cup chopped fresh parsley	
½ cup chopped fresh mint	4 cups baby spinach, divided

1. With a grater or food processor, grate the broccoli into grain-size pieces until it resembles rice. 2. Repeat with the jicama. You should have about 1 cup. 3. To a large bowl, add the grated broccoli, grated jicama, chickpeas, tomatoes, cucumber, parsley, mint, red onion, lemon juice, sunflower seeds, and olive oil. Toss until well mixed. Season with salt and pepper. 4. Arrange 2 cups of spinach on each of 2 plates. 5. Top each with half of the tabouli mixture. 6. Serve immediately.

Per Serving:

calorie: 265 | fat: 8g | protein: 9g | carbs: 44g | sugars: 10g | fiber: 21g | sodium: 138mg

Grilled Hearts of Romaine with Buttermilk Dressing

Prep time: 5 minutes | Cook time: 5 minutes | Serves 4

For The Romaine

2 heads romaine lettuce, halved lengthwise

2 tablespoons extra-virgin olive oil

For The Dressing

½ cup low-fat buttermilk

1 tablespoon extra-virgin olive oil

1 garlic clove, pressed

¼ bunch fresh chives, thinly chopped

1 pinch red pepper flakes

To Make The Romaine 1. Heat a grill pan over medium heat. 2. Brush each lettuce half with the olive oil, and place flat-side down on the grill. Grill for 3 to 5 minutes, or until the lettuce slightly wilts and develops light grill marks. To Make The Dressing 1. In a small bowl, whisk the buttermilk, olive oil, garlic, chives, and red pepper flakes together. 2. Drizzle 2 tablespoons of dressing over each romaine half, and serve.

Per Serving:

calorie: 157 | fat: 11g | protein: 5g | carbs: 12g | sugars: 5g | fiber: 7g | sodium: 84mg

Broccoli Slaw Crab Salad

Prep time: 15 minutes | Cook time: 0 minutes | Serves 4

⅔ cup mayonnaise

1 tablespoon freshly squeezed lime juice

1 teaspoon minced garlic

½ teaspoon freshly ground black pepper

1 (16-ounce) package broccoli slaw

2 (6-ounce) cans crabmeat, drained and flaked

1 small onion, diced

2 large celery stalks, chopped

1 large red bell pepper, seeded and chopped

Chopped fresh parsley, for garnish

1. In a large bowl, whisk together the mayonnaise, lime juice, garlic, and pepper until smooth. 2. Add the broccoli slaw, crab meat, onion, celery, and bell pepper and mix until all the ingredients are coated. 3. Garnish with parsley.

Per Serving:

calorie: 279 | fat: 14g | protein: 26g | carbs: 13g | sugars: 3g | fiber: 2g | sodium: 572mg

Chapter 13
Desserts

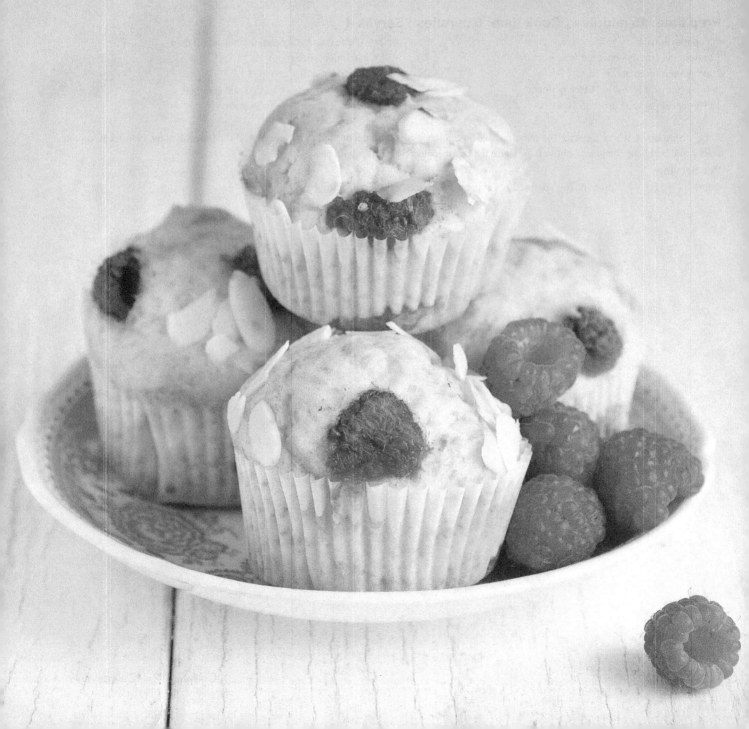

Peanut Butter Fudge Brownies

Prep time: 5 minutes | Cook time: 15 minutes | Makes 12 brownies

Cooking oil spray, as needed	1 teaspoon baking powder
1 cup (80 g) gluten-free rolled oats	¼ teaspoon sea salt
½ cup (48 g) almond flour	1 teaspoon ground cinnamon
1 cup (194 g) canned low-sodium black beans, drained and rinsed	⅓ cup (32 g) unsweetened cocoa powder
¼ cup (60 ml) cooking oil of choice	½ cup (120 ml) pure maple syrup
1½ teaspoon (8 ml) pure vanilla extract	¼ cup (45 g) dairy-free dark chocolate chips
¼ teaspoon baking soda	2 tablespoons (30 g) all-natural peanut butter (see Tip)

1. Preheat the oven to 350°F (177°C). Spray an 8 x 8–inch (20 x 20–cm) baking pan with the cooking oil spray. 2. In a food processor, combine the oats, almond flour, beans, oil, vanilla, baking soda, baking powder, sea salt, cinnamon, cocoa powder, and maple syrup. Process the ingredients for about 1 minute, until the batter is smooth. You may need to stop the food processor once and scrape down the sides. 3. Carefully remove the food processor's blade and stir in the chocolate chips by hand. 4. Spread the batter into the prepared baking pan. Drizzle the peanut butter over the top of the batter. 5. Bake the brownies for 15 minutes, until a toothpick inserted into the center comes out clean. Let the brownies cool completely in the pan on a wire rack.

Per Serving:
1 brownie: calorie: 170 | fat: 10g | protein: 3g | carbs: 19g | sugars: 11g | fiber: 2g | sodium: 52mg

Cherry Almond Cobbler

Prep time: 10 minutes | Cook time: 25 minutes | Serves 4

2 cups water-packed sour cherries	¾ teaspoon baking powder
¼ teaspoon fresh lemon juice	1 tablespoon canola oil
⅛ teaspoon almond extract	¼ cup egg substitute
½ cup almond flour, sifted	2 tablespoons fat-free milk
⅛ teaspoon salt	¼ cup granulated sugar substitute (such as stevia)
¼ cup flaxseeds	

1. Preheat the oven to 425 degrees. Drain the cherries, reserving ⅔ cup of liquid, and place the cherries in a shallow 9-inch glass or porcelain cake pan. 2. In a small mixing bowl, combine the lemon juice, almond extract, and drained cherry liquid; mix well. Spoon over the cherries. 3. In a mixing bowl, combine the almond flour, flaxseeds, and baking powder. Mix thoroughly. Stir in the oil, egg substitute, milk, and sugar substitute, mixing well. 4. Spoon the mixture over the cherries, and bake at 425 degrees for 25–30 minutes or until the crust is golden brown.

Per Serving:
calories: 216 | fat: 14g | protein: 7g | carbs: 19g | sugars: 10g | fiber: 6g | sodium: 132mg

Grilled Peach and Coconut Yogurt Bowls

Prep time: 5 minutes | Cook time: 10 minutes | Serves 4

2 peaches, halved and pitted	coconut flakes
½ cup plain nonfat Greek yogurt	2 tablespoons unsalted pistachios, shelled and broken into pieces
1 teaspoon pure vanilla extract	
¼ cup unsweetened dried	

1. Preheat the broiler to high. Arrange the rack in the closest position to the broiler. 2. In a shallow pan, arrange the peach halves, cut-side up. Broil for 6 to 8 minutes until browned, tender, and hot. 3. In a small bowl, mix the yogurt and vanilla. 4. Spoon the yogurt into the cavity of each peach half. 5. Sprinkle 1 tablespoon of coconut flakes and 1½ teaspoons of pistachios over each peach half. Serve warm.

Per Serving:
calories: 102 | fat: 5g | protein: 5g | carbs: 11g | sugars: 8g | fiber: 2g | sodium: 12mg

Chipotle Black Bean Brownies

Prep time: 15 minutes | Cook time: 30 minutes | Serves 8

Nonstick cooking spray	⅓ cup honey
½ cup dark chocolate chips, divided	1 teaspoon vanilla extract
¾ cup cooked calypso beans or black beans	⅓ cup white wheat flour
½ cup extra-virgin olive oil	½ teaspoon chipotle chili powder
2 large eggs	½ teaspoon ground cinnamon
¼ cup unsweetened dark chocolate cocoa powder	½ teaspoon baking powder
	½ teaspoon kosher salt

1. Spray a 7-inch Bundt pan with nonstick cooking spray. 2. Place half of the chocolate chips in a small bowl and microwave them for 30 seconds. Stir and repeat, if necessary, until the chips have completely melted. 3. In a food processor, blend the beans and oil together. Add the melted chocolate chips, eggs, cocoa powder, honey, and vanilla. Blend until the mixture is smooth. 4. In a large bowl, whisk together the flour, chili powder, cinnamon, baking powder, and salt. Pour the bean mixture from the food processor into the bowl and stir with a wooden spoon until well combined. Stir in the remaining chocolate chips. 5. Pour the batter into the prepared Bundt pan. Cover loosely with foil. 6. Pour 1 cup of water into the electric pressure cooker. 7. Place the Bundt pan onto the wire rack and lower it into the pressure cooker. 8. Close and lock the lid of the pressure cooker. Set the valve to sealing. 9. Cook on high pressure for 30 minutes. 10. When the cooking is complete, hit Cancel and quick release the pressure. 11. Once the pin drops, unlock and remove the lid. 12. Carefully transfer the pan to a cooling rack for about 10 minutes, then invert the cake onto the rack and let it cool completely. 13. Cut into slices and serve.

Per Serving:
(1 slice): calories: 296 | fat: 20g | protein: 5g | carbs: 29g | sugars: 16g | fiber: 4g | sodium: 224mg

Creamy Pineapple-Pecan Dessert Squares

Prep time: 25 minutes | Cook time: 0 minutes | Serves 18

¾ cup boiling water
1 package (4-serving size) lemon sugar-free gelatin
1 cup unsweetened pineapple juice
1½ cups graham cracker crumbs
½ cup sugar
¼ cup shredded coconut
¼ cup chopped pecans

3 tablespoons butter or margarine, melted
1 package (8 oz) fat-free cream cheese
1 container (8 oz) fat-free sour cream
1 can (8 oz) crushed pineapple, undrained

1 In large bowl, pour boiling water over gelatin; stir about 2 minutes or until gelatin is completely dissolved. Stir in pineapple juice. Refrigerate about 30 minutes or until mixture is syrupy and just beginning to thicken. 2 Meanwhile, in 13x9-inch (3-quart) glass baking dish, toss cracker crumbs, ¼ cup of the sugar, the coconut, pecans and melted butter until well mixed. Reserve ½ cup crumb mixture for topping. Press remaining mixture in bottom of dish. 3 In medium bowl, beat cream cheese, sour cream and remaining ¼ cup sugar with electric mixer on medium speed until smooth; set aside. 4 Beat gelatin mixture with electric mixer on low speed until foamy; beat on high speed until light and fluffy (mixture will look like beaten egg whites). Beat in cream cheese mixture just until mixed. Gently stir in pineapple (with liquid). Pour into crust-lined dish; smooth top. Sprinkle reserved ½ cup crumb mixture over top. Refrigerate about 4 hours or until set. For servings, cut into 6 rows by 3 rows.

Per Serving:
calorie: 120 | fat: 5g | protein: 3g | carbs: 18g | sugars: 11g | fiber: 0g | sodium: 180mg

Mango Nice Cream

Prep time: 10 minutes | Cook time: 0 minutes | Serves 4

2 cups frozen mango chunks
1 cup frozen, sliced, overripe banana (can use room temperature, but must be overripe)
Pinch of sea salt

½ teaspoon pure vanilla extract
¼ cup and 1 to 2 tablespoons low-fat nondairy milk
2 to 3 tablespoons coconut nectar or pure maple syrup (optional)

1. In a food processor or high-speed blender, combine the mango, banana, salt, vanilla, and ¼ cup of the milk. Pulse to get things moving, and then puree, adding the remaining 1 to 2 tablespoons milk if needed. Taste, and add the nectar or syrup, if desired. Serve, or transfer to an airtight container and freeze for an hour or more to set more firmly before serving.

Per Serving:
calorie: 116 | fat: 1g | protein: 1g | carbs: 29g | sugars: 22g | fiber: 2g | sodium: 81mg

Superfood Brownie Bites

Prep time: 15 minutes | Cook time: 0 minutes | Makes 30

1 cup raw nuts (walnuts, pecans, or cashews)
½ cup hulled hemp seeds
⅓ cup raw pepitas

½ cup raw cacao powder
1 cup pitted dates
2 tablespoons coconut oil
1 teaspoon vanilla extract

1. Line a baking sheet with parchment paper. 2. Place the nuts, hemp seeds, and pepitas in a food processor and pulse until the ingredients are a meal consistency. Add the cacao powder, dates, coconut oil, and vanilla extract and pulse until the mixture holds together if you pinch it with your fingers. The dough should ball up and appear glossy, and not be too sticky and wet. If it doesn't stick together enough to form a dough consistency, add water in drops until the correct consistency is reached. Be careful not to add too much liquid. If you do, add more cacao to balance the texture. 3. Scoop out the brownie bite mixture in 1-tablespoon amounts and roll the mixture into balls. Set the balls on the baking sheet and then chill them in the refrigerator for at least 10 minutes to hold their shape. 4. Transfer the balls to a container with a lid and store in the refrigerator until ready to eat. You could eat these immediately, but they are more likely to crumble. 5. Store brownies in an airtight container in the refrigerator for 5 to 7 days.

Per Serving:
calories: 145 | fat: 11g | protein: 4g | carbs: 11g | sugars: 7g | fiber: 3g | sodium: 2mg

Oatmeal Chippers

Prep time: 10 minutes | Cook time: 11 minutes | Makes 20 chippers

3 to 3½ tablespoons almond butter (or tigernut butter, for nut-free)
¼ cup pure maple syrup
¼ cup brown rice syrup
2 teaspoons pure vanilla extract
1⅓ cups oat flour

1 cup + 2 tablespoons rolled oats
1½ teaspoons baking powder
½ teaspoon cinnamon
¼ teaspoon sea salt
2 to 3 tablespoons sugar-free nondairy chocolate chips

1. Preheat the oven to 350°F. Line a baking sheet with parchment paper. 2. In the bowl of a mixer, combine the almond butter, maple syrup, brown rice syrup, and vanilla. Using the paddle attachment, mix on low speed for a couple of minutes, until creamy. Turn off the mixer and add the flour, oats, baking powder, cinnamon, salt, and chocolate chips. Mix on low speed until incorporated. Place 1½-tablespoon mounds on the prepared baking sheet, spacing them 1" to 2" apart, and flatten slightly. Bake for 11 minutes, or until just set to the touch. Remove from the oven, let cool on the pan for just a minute, and then transfer the cookies to a cooling rack.

Per Serving:
calorie: 90 | fat: 2g | protein: 2g | carbs: 16g | sugars: 4g | fiber: 2g | sodium: 75mg

Strawberry Cheesecake in a Jar

Prep time: 5 minutes | Cook time: 0 minutes | Serves 8

½ cup (55 g) raw cashews
¼ cup (60 g) all-natural peanut butter
2 tablespoons (12 g) almond flour
1 large pitted Medjool date
1 cup (200 g) coarsely chopped strawberries, plus more as needed

8 ounces (227 g) cream cheese
½ cup (100 g) plain nonfat Greek yogurt
¼ cup (60 ml) pure maple syrup
Zest of 1 medium lemon, plus more as needed
1 tablespoon (15 ml) pure vanilla extract

1. In a food processor, combine the cashews, peanut butter, almond flour, and Medjool date. Process the ingredients until a dough forms. 2. Divide the dough among eight (8 ounces [227 ml]) mason jars. Press the dough down into each jar to make a crust. 3. Divide the strawberries among the jars on top of the crusts. 4. In a food processor or high power blender, combine the cream cheese, yogurt, maple syrup, lemon zest, and vanilla. Process the ingredients until they are smooth. 5. Divide the cheesecake mixture evenly among the jars, tapping them gently on the counter to shake out all the air bubbles. 6. Top the cheesecakes with additional strawberries and lemon zest if desired. 7. Refrigerate the cheesecakes for at least 2 hours or overnight before serving.

Per Serving:

calorie: 253 | fat: 18g | protein: 7g | carbs: 17g | sugars: 12g | fiber: 2g | sodium: 115mg

Mixed-Berry Cream Tart

Prep time: 20 minutes | Cook time: 0 minutes | Serves 8

2 cups sliced fresh strawberries
½ cup boiling water
1 box (4-serving size) sugar-free strawberry gelatin
3 pouches (1½ ounces each) roasted almond crunchy granola bars (from 8.9-oz box)
1 package (8 ounces) fat-free

cream cheese
¼ cup sugar
¼ teaspoon almond extract
1 cup fresh blueberries
1 cup fresh raspberries
Fat-free whipped topping, if desired

1. In small bowl, crush 1 cup of the strawberries with pastry blender or fork. Reserve remaining 1 cup strawberries. 2. In medium bowl, pour boiling water over gelatin; stir about 2 minutes or until gelatin is completely dissolved. Stir crushed strawberries into gelatin. Refrigerate 20 minutes. 3. Meanwhile, leaving granola bars in pouches, crush granola bars with rolling pin. Sprinkle crushed granola in bottom of 9-inch ungreased glass pie plate, pushing crumbs up side of plate to make crust. 4. In small bowl, beat cream cheese, sugar and almond extract with electric mixer on medium-high speed until smooth. Drop by spoonfuls over crushed granola; gently spread to cover bottom of crust. 5. Gently fold blueberries, raspberries and remaining 1 cup strawberries into gelatin mixture. Spoon over cream cheese mixture. Refrigerate about 3 hours or until

firm. Serve topped with whipped topping.

Per Serving:

calorie: 170 | fat: 3g | protein: 8g | carbs: 27g | sugars: 17g | fiber: 3g | sodium: 340mg

Blackberry Yogurt Ice Pops

Prep time: 10 minutes | Cook time: 0 minutes | Serves 4

12 ounces plain Greek yogurt
1 cup blackberries
Pinch nutmeg

¼ cup milk
2 (1-gram) packets stevia

1. In a blender, combine all of the ingredients. Blend until smooth. 2. Pour the mixture into 4 ice pop molds. Freeze for 6 hours before serving.

Per Serving:

calories: 71 | fat: 1g | protein: 10g | carbs: 8g | sugars: 5g | fiber: 2g | sodium: 37mg

Berry Smoothie Pops

Prep time: 5 minutes | Cook time: 0 minutes | Serves 6

2 cups frozen mixed berries
½ cup unsweetened plain almond milk

1 cup plain nonfat Greek yogurt
2 tablespoons hemp seeds

1. Place all the ingredients in a blender and process until finely blended. 2. Pour into 6 clean ice pop molds and insert sticks. 3. Freeze for 3 to 4 hours until firm.

Per Serving:

calorie: 70 | fat: 2g | protein: 5g | carbs: 9g | sugars: 2g | fiber: 3g | sodium: 28mg

Baked Pumpkin Pudding

Prep time: 5 minutes | Cook time: 20 minutes | Serves 4

1½ cups mashed pumpkin
1 egg
2½ tablespoons agave nectar
½ teaspoon vanilla extract

1 teaspoon pumpkin pie spice
¼ cup slivered almonds
¼ cup raisins

1. Preheat the oven to 350 degrees. 2. In a large bowl, combine the pumpkin, egg, agave nectar, vanilla, and pumpkin pie spice, and mix well. Stir in the almonds and raisins, leaving a few for garnish. 3. Spoon the mixture into 4 ramekins, and garnish with the remaining almonds and raisins. 4. Bake at 350 degrees for approximately 20 minutes, or until golden on top. 5. Serve warm or at room temperature.

Per Serving:

calories: 130 | fat: 5g | protein: 4g | carbs: 20g | sugars: 13g | fiber: 2g | sodium: 18mg

Low-Calorie, Fat-Free Whipped Cream

Prep time: 5 minutes | Cook time: 5 minutes | Serves 8

2 tablespoons water	1 teaspoon vanilla extract
1 teaspoon unflavored gelatin	1 cup ice water
½ cup fat-free powdered milk	½ teaspoon agave nectar

1. In a small skillet, add the water; sprinkle gelatin on top. 2. After the gelatin has soaked in, stir over low heat until clear; cool. In a large mixing bowl, combine the milk, vanilla, ice water, and agave nectar; mix well. 3. Add the gelatin mixture, and whip until fluffy with a wire whisk or electric beaters. Refrigerate the whipped cream until ready to use.

Per Serving:
calories: 10 | fat: 0g | protein: 1g | carbs: 1g | sugars: 1g | fiber: 0g | sodium: 11mg

Blender Banana Snack Cake

Prep time: 5 minutes | Cook time: 30 to 32 minutes | Serves 9

¼ cup coconut nectar or pure maple syrup	¼ teaspoon sea salt
¼ cup water	3½ cups sliced, well-ripened bananas
2 teaspoons vanilla	1 cup whole grain spelt flour
1 teaspoon cinnamon	½ cup rolled oats
½ teaspoon nutmeg	2 teaspoons baking powder

1. Preheat the oven to 350°F. Lightly coat an 8" x 8" pan with cooking spray and line the bottom of the pan with parchment paper. 2. In a blender, combine the nectar or syrup, water, vanilla, cinnamon, nutmeg, salt, and 3 cups of the sliced bananas. Puree until smooth. Add the flour, oats, baking powder, and the remaining ½ cup of bananas. Pulse a couple of times, until just combined. (Don't puree; you don't want to overwork the flour.) Transfer the mixture into the baking dish, using a spatula to scrape down the sides of the bowl. Bake for 30 to 32 minutes, until fully set. (Insert a toothpick in the center and see if it comes out clean.) Transfer the cake pan to a cooling rack. Let cool completely before cutting.

Per Serving:
calorie: 141 | fat: 1g | protein: 3g | carbs: 32g | sugars: 14g | fiber: 4g | sodium: 177mg

Pineapple-Peanut Nice Cream

Prep time: 10 minutes | Cook time: 0 minutes | Serves 6

2 cups frozen pineapple	½ cup unsweetened almond milk
1 cup peanut butter (no added sugar, salt, or fat)	

1. In a blender or food processor, combine the frozen pineapple and peanut butter and process. 2. Add the almond milk, and blend until smooth. The end result should be a smooth paste.

Per Serving:
calories: 143 | fat: 3g | protein: 10g | carbs: 15g | sugars: 7g | fiber: 3g | sodium: 22mg

Dark Chocolate–Cherry Multigrain Cookies

Prep time: 40 minutes | Cook time: 7 to 8 minutes | Makes 18 cookies

½ cup packed brown sugar	¾ cup uncooked 5-grain rolled hot cereal
3 tablespoons granulated sugar	½ teaspoon baking soda
⅓ cup canola oil	¼ teaspoon salt
1 egg or ¼ cup fat-free egg product	½ cup dried cherries
2 teaspoons vanilla	⅓ cup bittersweet chocolate chips
1 cup white whole wheat flour	

1. Heat oven to 375°F. In medium bowl, mix sugars, oil, egg and vanilla. Stir in flour, cereal, baking soda and salt until blended (dough will be slightly soft). Stir in cherries and chocolate chips. 2. Onto ungreased cookie sheets, drop dough by rounded tablespoonfuls 2 inches apart. Bake 7 to 8 minutes or until light golden brown around edges (centers will look slightly underdone). Cool 1 minute; transfer from cookie sheets to cooling racks. Cool completely.

Per Serving:
1 Cookie: calorie: 160 | fat: 6g | protein: 2g | carbs: 23g | sugars: 13g | fiber: 2g | sodium: 110mg

Banana Pudding

Prep time: 30 minutes | Cook time: 20 minutes | Serves 10

For The Pudding	2 (8-ounce) containers sugar-free spelt hazelnut biscuits, crushed
¾ cup erythritol or other sugar replacement	5 medium bananas, sliced
5 teaspoons almond flour	For The Meringue
¼ teaspoon salt	5 medium egg whites (1 cup)
2½ cups fat-free milk	¼ cup erythritol or other sugar replacement
6 tablespoons prepared egg replacement	½ teaspoon vanilla extract
½ teaspoon vanilla extract	

Make The Pudding: 1. In a saucepan, whisk the erythritol, almond flour, salt, and milk together. Cook over medium heat until the sugar is dissolved. 2. Whisk in the egg replacement and cook for about 10 minutes, or until thickened. 3. Remove from the heat and stir in the vanilla. 4. Spread the thickened pudding onto the bottom of a 3 × 6-inch casserole dish. 5. Arrange a layer of crushed biscuits on top of the pudding. 6. Place a layer of sliced bananas on top of the biscuits. Make The Meringue: 1. Preheat the oven to 350°F. 2. In a medium bowl, beat the egg whites for about 5 minutes, or until stiff. 3. Add the erythritol and vanilla while continuing to beat for about 3 more minutes. 4. Spread the meringue on top of the banana pudding. 5. Transfer the casserole dish to the oven, and bake for 7 to 10 minutes, or until the top is lightly browned.

Per Serving:
calories: 323 | fat: 14g | protein: 12g | carbs: 42g | sugars: 11g | fiber: 3g | sodium: 148mg

Avocado Chocolate Mousse

Prep time: 5 minutes | Cook time: 0 minutes | Serves 4

2 avocados, mashed

¼ cup canned coconut milk

2 tablespoons unsweetened cocoa powder

2 tablespoons pure maple syrup

½ teaspoon espresso powder

½ teaspoon vanilla extract

1. In a blender, combine all of the ingredients. Blend until smooth. 2. Pour the mixture into 4 small bowls and serve.

Per Serving:

calories: 222 | fat: 18g | protein: 3g | carbs: 17g | sugars: 7g | fiber: 8g | sodium: 11mg

Grilled Watermelon with Avocado Mousse

Prep time: 10 minutes | Cook time: 10 minutes | Serves 8

1 small, seedless watermelon, halved and cut into 1-inch rounds

2 ripe avocados, pitted and

peeled

½ cup fat-free plain yogurt

¼ teaspoon cayenne pepper

1. On a hot grill, grill the watermelon slices for 2 to 3 minutes on each side, or until you can see the grill marks. 2. To make the avocado mousse, in a blender, combine the avocados, yogurt, and cayenne and process until smooth. 3. To serve, cut each watermelon round in half. Top each with a generous dollop of avocado mousse.

Per Serving:

calories: 162 | fat: 8g | protein: 3g | carbs: 22g | sugars: 14g | fiber: 5g | sodium: 13mg

Banana Pineapple Freeze

Prep time: 30 minutes | Cook time: 0 minutes | Serves 12

2 cups mashed ripe bananas

2 cups unsweetened orange juice

2 tablespoon fresh lemon juice

1 cup unsweetened crushed pineapple, undrained

½ teaspoon ground cinnamon

1. In a food processor, combine all ingredients, and process until smooth and creamy. 2. Pour the mixture into a 9-x-9-x-2-inch baking dish, and freeze overnight or until firm. Serve chilled.

Per Serving:

calories: 60 | fat: 0g | protein: 1g | carbs: 15g | sugars: 9g | fiber: 1g | sodium: 1mg

Dulce de Leche Fillo Cups

Prep time: 15 minutes | Cook time: 0 minutes | Serves 15

2 ounces ⅓-less-fat cream cheese (Neufchâtel), softened

2 tablespoons dulce de leche (caramel) syrup

1 tablespoon reduced-fat sour

cream

1 package frozen mini fillo shells (15 shells)

⅓ cup sliced fresh strawberries

2 tablespoons diced mango

1. In medium bowl, beat cream cheese with electric mixer on low speed until creamy. Beat in dulce de leche syrup and sour cream until blended. 2. Spoon cream cheese mixture into each fillo shell. Top each with strawberries and mango.

Per Serving:

calorie: 40 | fat: 2g | protein: 0g | carbs: 4g | sugars: 2g | fiber: 0g | sodium: 35mg

Appendix 1:

Measurement Conversion Chart

VOLUME EQUIVALENTS(DRY)

US STANDARD	METRIC (APPROXIMATE)
1/8 teaspoon	0.5 mL
1/4 teaspoon	1 mL
1/2 teaspoon	2 mL
3/4 teaspoon	4 mL
1 teaspoon	5 mL
1 tablespoon	15 mL
1/4 cup	59 mL
1/2 cup	118 mL
3/4 cup	177 mL
1 cup	235 mL
2 cups	475 mL
3 cups	700 mL
4 cups	1 L

WEIGHT EQUIVALENTS

US STANDARD	METRIC (APPROXIMATE)
1 ounce	28 g
2 ounces	57 g
5 ounces	142 g
10 ounces	284 g
15 ounces	425 g
16 ounces (1 pound)	455 g
1.5 pounds	680 g
2 pounds	907 g

VOLUME EQUIVALENTS(LIQUID)

US STANDARD	US STANDARD (OUNCES)	METRIC (APPROXIMATE)
2 tablespoons	1 fl.oz.	30 mL
1/4 cup	2 fl.oz.	60 mL
1/2 cup	4 fl.oz.	120 mL
1 cup	8 fl.oz.	240 mL
1 1/2 cup	12 fl.oz.	355 mL
2 cups or 1 pint	16 fl.oz.	475 mL
4 cups or 1 quart	32 fl.oz.	1 L
1 gallon	128 fl.oz.	4 L

TEMPERATURES EQUIVALENTS

FAHRENHEIT(F)	CELSIUS(C) (APPROXIMATE)
225 °F	107 °C
250 °F	120 °C
275 °F	135 °C
300 °F	150 °C
325 °F	160 °C
350 °F	180 °C
375 °F	190 °C
400 °F	205 °C
425 °F	220 °C
450 °F	235 °C
475 °F	245 °C
500 °F	260 °C

Appendix 2:

The Dirty Dozen and Clean Fifteen

The Environmental Working Group (EWG) is a nonprofit, nonpartisan organization dedicated to protecting human health and the environment Its mission is to empower people to live healthier lives in a healthier environment. This organization publishes an annual list of the twelve kinds of produce, in sequence, that have the highest amount of pesticide residue-the Dirty Dozen-as well as a list of the fifteen kinds ofproduce that have the least amount of pesticide residue-the Clean Fifteen.

THE DIRTY DOZEN	THE CLEAN FIFTEEN
• The 2016 Dirty Dozen includes the following produce. These are considered among the year's most important produce to buy organic:	• The least critical to buy organically are the Clean Fifteen list. The following are on the 2016 list:

Strawberries	Spinach	Avocados	Papayas
Apples	Tomatoes	Corn	Kiw
Nectarines	Bell peppers	Pineapples	Eggplant
Peaches	Cherry tomatoes	Cabbage	Honeydew
Celery	Cucumbers	Sweet peas	Grapefruit
Grapes	Kale/collard greens	Onions	Cantaloupe
Cherries	Hot peppers	Asparagus	Cauliflower
		Mangos	

• *The Dirty Dozen list contains two additional itemskale/collard greens and hot peppers-because they tend to contain trace levels of highly hazardous pesticides.*

• *Some of the sweet corn sold in the United States are made from genetically engineered (GE) seedstock. Buy organic varieties of these crops to avoid GE produce.*

Appendix 3:

Recipe Index

Made in the USA
Las Vegas, NV
19 February 2024